The Inflammation Solution

Dr. Sears Wellness Books

Prime-Time Health
The Omega-3 Effect
Natural Astaxanthin – Hawaii's Supernutrient

Dr. Sears Parenting Library

The A.D.D. Book
The Allergy Book
The Attachment Parenting Book
The Autism Book
The Baby Book
The Baby Sleep Book
The Birth Book
The Breastfeeding Book
The Discipline Book
The Family Nutrition Book
The Fussy Baby Book
The Healthiest Kid in the Neighborhood
The Healthy Pregnancy Book
The N.D.D. Book
The Portable Pediatrician
The Pregnancy Book
The Premature Baby Book
The Successful Child Book
The Vaccine Book

Dr. Sears Children's Library

Baby on the Way
Eat Healthy, Feel Great
What Baby Needs
You Can Go to the Potty

THE INFLAMMATION SOLUTION

When Everything Works and Nothing Hurts

William Sears, M.D.
Foreword by Vincent Fortanasce, M.D.

Dr. Sears Wellness Institute Library

Dr. Sears Wellness Institute
384 Inverness Parkway
Englewood, Colorado 80112

First Edition: April 2015

Illustrations by Debbie Maze

ISBN 978-0-9962664-0-6

Printed in the United States of America

To our children, I wish to leave you the legacy of good health:

James

Robert

Peter

Hayden

Erin

Matthew

Stephen

Lauren

*To my wife, Martha, may this Inflammation Solution
keep me part of your life for many more years.*

TABLE OF CONTENTS

Chapter 3: Twelve Simple Ways to Eat the Anti-Inflammatory Way 116

Chapter 4: Move to Your Inflammation's Content 144

Chapter 5: Reduce Your Waist 163

Chapter 6: Don't Worry, Be Less Inflamed 170

Chapter 7: Self-help for the ABCDs: *A*rthritis, *B*ronchitis, *C*olitis, *C*ognitivitis, and *D*ermatitis 190

Chapter 8: The Inflammation Solution Begins At Birth 245

FOREWORD

Dr. William Sears' book, *The Inflammation Solution,* is a sincere and straightforward message of the power we have over our health and well-being in an age where the American lifestyle – sedentary, stressful, with a diet full of refined carbohydrates – has become our greatest health hazard.

It is a great honor to have Dr. Sears as a colleague. I could use the words erudite and sagacious to describe him, but Dr. Sears' greatest skills are making the complex simple, science understandable, and the impossible possible. So, I describe him with the words insightful, intelligent, and compassionate.

The field of holistic medicine, the mixture of Eastern "natural and nurturing" with Western "mechanical and pharmaceutical," is taking root in the United States. Dr. Sears takes the best of both worlds and combines them in *The Inflammation Solution.* It is a book of self-empowerment that helps you, the reader, realize you are in control of your body, your mind, and your health.

Last year the *New England Journal of Medicine* declared that neurological degenerative diseases, such as Alzheimer's, are the number one diagnosed illnesses today, more common than heart disease and cancer. Deaths from neurodegenerative diseases are up 69 percent, whereas heart and cancer deaths are down.

The bad news is, as the American Neurological Association has predicted, 40 percent of the 78 million baby-boomers born between 1946 and 1964 will get Alzheimer's disease. We are at the doorstep of a medical calamity. The primary cause, both Eastern and Western medicine agree, is inflammation and oxidative stress.

The good news is they both can be eliminated. The best news is *The Inflammation Solution* can give you the tools and methodology to start today before it is too late. Studies have shown that these methods are effective no matter what age you start. The secret of success is to begin today!

Remember, modern medicine has increased our lifespan, but has not increased our brain-span. Dr. Sears' revolutionary ideas do what pharmaceutical medicine does not. He gets to the root of and prescribes the changes in lifestyle that prevent these degenerative diseases.

– Vincent Fortanasce, M.D.
Clinical and associate professor of neurology at the University of Southern California and author of *The Anti-Alzheimer's Prescription* and *End Back & Neck Pain.*

DR. BILL'S HEALING NOTE TO READERS

My health wish for you: everything works and nothing hurts! *The Inflammation Solution* is a timely text for all organs and all ages. Once upon a time, "doctor" meant "teacher." Now it means "prescriber." The medical model of patient care that I have practiced for over 40 years is what I call the pills-and-skills model. When a person comes into my office complaining of an "-itis" illness, I often prescribe pills for the illness, but also give my patients a list of self-help skills. The skill-teaching usually takes more time than scribbling out a prescription for the pills. I teach my patients: "Here's what you *take*, and here's what you *do.*"

Due to changes in healthcare, dubbed volume-oriented medicine, a doctor is now economically pushed into being a pill-pusher instead of a skill-teacher. Reimbursement to doctors is going down, yet the cost of running a medical practice is going up. Obvious solution: see more patients per unit of time! And it takes much less time to prescribe pills than to teach skills. Especially for inflammatory illnesses, the best answer to this current model of healthcare is *self-care*. For a person with any inflammatory illness, it begins with this book.

I'm a show-me-the-science doctor. I won't put anything in my books or prescribe any medicine in my medical practice that is not backed up by solid science. That is my promise to you, my readers. The Inflammation Solution Plan that you read, do, and feel is backed up by solid science, years of practical experience, and given the stamp of approval by my trusted board of advisors – those experts in inflammatory illnesses that you will meet in the resources section on page 267.

Among my medical colleagues, I'm known as the science-made-simple doctor. Learning about inflammatory illnesses can read like a confusing college course in biochemistry, so throughout the book I've tried to use the KISMIF principle: Keep It Simple, Make It Fun. You will also be treated to lots of wise one-liners from my "partner" in medical practice, Dr. Feelbetter, who specializes in solving your inflammation problems. Our prescription: Read it, do it, feel it.

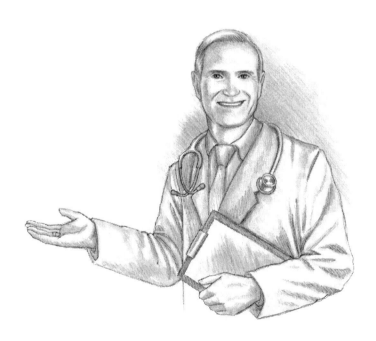

PART I

THE INFLAMMATION PROBLEM

Have you noticed the news lately? "We are an inflammation nation." "The U.S. is on fire." "Americans spend more on painkiller medicines than any other country." "Inflammation, the silent killer." Welcome to the inflame-age.

PAINFUL STATISTICS

Consider these effects of "-itis" illnesses on our healthcare system:

- As of 2012, 52 million Americans suffer from some form of arthritis.
- Patients spend over 20 billion dollars a year on anti-inflammatory drugs.
- Inflammatory illnesses are collectively the most common reason for hospitalization and seeking medical treatment.
- Arthritis is the number one cause of chronic pain and affects over 30 percent of adults.
- Inflammatory illnesses are the number one cause of disabilities.
- Inflammatory illnesses are the number one cause of premature and unhealthy aging.
- Anti-inflammatory drugs top the list of medicines having undesirable side effects.

As you read, you will learn the healthful concept of *inflammation balance*: A body in balance heals. A body out of balance hurts. First, I want you to understand how your body is remarkably designed to heal and what you may be doing to sabotage this natural process. Once you realize why you have pain going on inside your body, in Part II we'll look at some solutions.

PREVENT INFLAMMATION PROBLEMS

In most inflammatory illnesses, such as arthritis, by the time you feel it the body takes a long time to heal it. In case you already have "silent" inflammation going on inside your body, get in the "prevent" mode, rather than the "repair" mode. Doctor's orders!

CHAPTER 1

What "-itis" Is In Your Body?

We all want mobility without pain and remedies without harm. If you suffer from inflammation, this book is your solution. Inflammation is the number one cause of illness and aging; yet it is the most preventable and treatable cause. Inflammation is the main reason that people have the three Ds: disease, disabilities, and doctors' visits. In fact, most of a doctor's day in the medical office is spent treating the ABCDs: *a*rthritis, *b*ronchitis, *c*olitis, *c*ognitivitis and *d*ermatitis. Nearly every illness from head-to-toe has its roots in inflammation:

- Cognitiv*itis* (Alzheimer's)
- Gingiv*itis* (gum disease)
- Card*itis* (cardiovascular disease)
- Bronch*itis* (asthma)
- Col*itis* (intestinal illnesses)
- Dermat*itis* (skin inflammation)
- Arthr*itis* (joint pains)
- Nephr*itis* (kidney disease)
- Retin*itis* (vision loss)

And, in the last decade more "-itis" illnesses are filling doctors' offices:

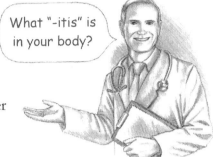

What "-itis" is in your body?

- Thyroid*itis*
- Endothelial*itis* (clots in blood vessels)
- Postur*itis* (hunching over high-tech gadgets)

In addition, you may be surprised to learn that autism may be in the spectrum of an autoimmune disease whereby the child's own immune system attacks certain areas in the brain. Increasing research is starting to support this correlation.

THE PROBLEM: WHY WE HURT

Do you ever wonder why we get inflamed? The term "inflammation" means "on fire." Americans are the most inflamed people in the world. Call us the inflammation nation. Americans are "on fire," but with illness, not with health. We need to know how the fire starts and what preventive-medicine fire extinguishers to use. Inflammation itself is good. It's a healthy part of metabolism and healing. It's a normal response by your body's department of defense – your immune system. It is vital to your survival.

The inflammatory response is one of the oldest survival mechanisms. Designed to protect, repair, and heal, we could not live without it. That is why the body's entry points for germs and collection points for toxins (the lining of skin, breathing passages, gut, blood vessels, and joints) are equipped with powerful resident armies. These are the tissues most prone to battle damage, or "-itis". In these areas, the "good inflammation" that heals us can turn into "bad inflammation" that hurts us.

Excess inflammation is too much of a good thing. There's a constant fight, or fire, going on inside your body. Your immune system army is constantly on a search-and-destroy mission. Each soldier, or immune biochemical, is programmed to identify agents that enter your body. Your immune soldiers identify healthy foods, clean air, and harmless bacteria as "self," that is, "You are friendly and belong in this body, so I will leave you alone." And they identify as "non-self", or alien, such things as germs, junk food, unhealthy biochemicals and toxins, concluding: "You are foreign and don't belong here, so we're going to attack you, fight you, and get rid of you so you don't harm the body." Sounds healthy, and it is, up to a point.

The case of the cut finger. When the immune system soldiers fight the germ, a mini "fire" breaks out, hence the term "inflammation," or in this case "friendly fire." For example, you cut your finger, and germs get under the skin. Inflammatory soldiers rush to the scene of the crime to prevent infection and tissue damage from the splinter. You start feeling the inflammatory effect of these tiny fires in your finger. The area gets red, swollen, and feels hot; and you may even notice "throbbing" as more blood flow comes to the site of the battle. (The bloodstream is the immune army's transport system.) That's the *inflammatory response* you see and feel in your finger. That's healthy inflammation, and the fighters are called *pro-inflammatories*, or fire starters.

Your body's social network. Just imagine millions of these microscopic soldiers traveling around your body. The communication commandos of the army are called *cytokines* ("cell movers"). Like cyto-texting or chemical emails, these biochemicals travel all over the body and send signals that germ invasion or disease is going on and the body needs help. Cytokines have obvious names, such as *interleukins* (messengers that talk between leukocytes, or white blood cells); and *interferons* (messengers that interfere with germs getting into tissues). These commandos mobilize the immune system army from the lymph nodes in the gut, the spleen, or wherever the nearest army is to the battleground. For example, if you have a cut, cytokines notify platelets and fibrin, which are like microscopic paramedics with bandages, to rush to the site of the hurt and stop the bleeding. These cytokines, or chemical messengers, go hunting for reinforcements, such as white blood cells, and attach themselves to these cell-soldiers, personally escorting them to the battlefield. A prominent cytokine that you all know, and have felt, is *histamine*, the biochemical that rushes to the entry of an allergen in the nasal membrane to flush it out. Then we sometimes take an antihistamine to dial it down when the nose continues to drip.

Remember me? The first job of your immune system is surveillance, differentiating between cells that are normal parts of the body and belong there, and cells or germs that are invaders. Immuno-speak is "self" and "non-self," or "belong here" and "don't belong here." The immune system possesses a vast memory. After it attacks an invading foreign cell, say a germ or chemical toxin, and destroys it, the army remembers what that cell looks like. If that cell tries to reenter, the body is then primed to get rid of it more quickly. This is the basis for vaccines, priming the immune system with a bit of the germ so it's ready for the big fight when the real germ appears.

Meet the troops. The two key players on your immune team, antibodies and white blood cells, are strategically located at checkpoints throughout your body, especially where germs are more likely to enter, such as the lungs, intestines, and bloodstream. Think of the three types of fighter immune cells – T-cells from the thymus, B-cells from the bone marrow, and natural killer (NK) cells – like military bases. These military bases are constantly sending out radar signals to detect foreign germs that enter the body, and they try to remember those they've met before. After detecting the "terrorists," they send out antibodies called T-cells, which are *smart bombs*, to travel around the body to destroy the germs. The B-cells make specific antibodies that bind to the surface of the germ like a barcode stamp, targeting it for destruction by the immune cellular army. Finally, special white blood cells, called macrophages ("big eaters"), mop up the war zone and the body is back in inflammation balance. Much of this army's time is spent correctly identifying foreign germs, such as bacteria and viruses, and artificial chemical foods or fake foods dubbed "frankenfoods." The troops conclude: "You don't belong here. We're going to attack you."

How they fight and how they fail.   As if we need another dysfunction, inflammation imbalance could really be called "immune dysfunction."   First, the immune system army can entirely miss the invader. The germ gets through the checkpoints of the lungs, through the gut or skin into the bloodstream, and goes undetected until it causes harm or illness. Second, too many germs can enter the body

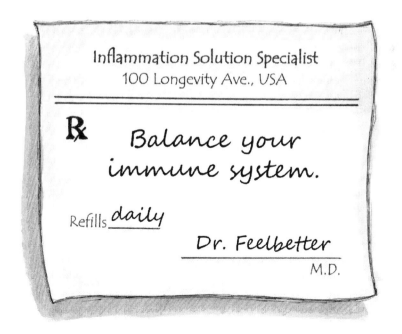

Inflammation Solution Specialist
100 Longevity Ave., USA

R̶x   Balance your
immune system.

Refills daily

Dr. Feelbetter

M.D.

too quickly and overwhelm the immune system. Take, for example, the flu. A big fight breaks out: fever, fatigue, and chills – all signs of inflammation, that your immune system is fighting the germs. After four or five days of flu-fighting, the immune system wins. You start feeling better because the battle is over. A third, different kind of fight is the worst one. Sometimes the immune system gets its signals mixed up, doesn't correctly identify self vs. non-self, and starts attacking the body's own tissues, mistaking them for foreigners, such as the lining of joints (arthritis), the lining of the gut (colitis), skin (dermatitis), and so on. These are called *autoimmune diseases*, meaning the immune system attacks itself, sort of like an army mistakenly attacking its own soldiers. Finally, sometimes the immune system is confused when a foreign invader, such as a factory-made chemical coloring,, attaches to part of a real food: "Do I attack the real food or the fake food or both?" Hence the epidemic of food allergies.

INFLAMMATION HEALTH MADE SIMPLE

- *Inflammation balance* means the "fire starters" (pro-inflammatory biochemicals) are balanced by the "fire extinguishers" (anti-inflammatory biochemicals).

- *Inflammation imbalance* means that inside your body you have more fires than fire extinguishers.

How "-itises" heal. Meanwhile, back at the sore finger, as the inflammation subsides, and the swelling, redness, and heat lessen, there is a mess left within the tissues like debris after a battle, known as "tissue wear and tear." So another group of soldiers, called anti-inflammatories – fire extinguishers – (I like to call them the healers) come into the tissues and repair them.

Throughout the book, I use the term "anti-inflammatory," but really the better term is "inflammation balance." Anti-inflammatory is like its misnomer cousin, "anti-aging." If you don't have the right amount of inflammation, your immune system shuts down, the germs overtake your body, and you get sick. You can guess what happens if you "anti-age". I also prefer the term immune system "balance" rather than immune system "boost." In some autoimmune illnesses, the immune system is boosted too strongly.

BODIES OUT OF BALANCE: A SECOND HELPING

To be sure you understand immune balance, let's go back into your body to see what could go wrong. Health, or wellness, occurs when your body enjoys *inflammation balance*, meaning wear and tear equals repair. Yet, after years of inflammatory battles, such as having to put out too many fires, the immune system armies harm and hurt rather than help and heal in these ways:

Over-inflammation. The wear and tear overwhelms the repair, leaving a lot of rough edges, say in the blood vessels, the lining of the gut, or in the joints. Sort of like biochemical stranger anxiety, the anti-inflammatory soldiers overreact and over-repair, such as potholes in a road being way overfilled, leading to a bumpy, rough road. Since most of the inflammatory fights occur in the entry and collection points of germs and toxins, like the front lines on the battlefield, chronic "-itis" illnesses begin in the lining tissues of the body: bronchitis, colitis, and arthritis.

Mistaken inflammation. Another way the body's inflammatory defense mechanism may go wrong is in a case of mistaken identity, as described on page 7. It may confuse the body's own tissue for an enemy and attack, such as at the lining of the joints (rheumatoid arthritis), the lining of the bowel (inflammatory bowel disease), and even the thyroid (thyroiditis). One root cause of the autoimmune disease epidemic is when you feed the immune system artificial food and you develop an artificial immune response.

Over-metabolism. Like a car engine burns fuel for energy, so your body burns food for energy, a combination of processes called metabolism. These normal fires of metabolism are called oxidants or *oxidation* (oxygen-burning). As you will later learn, when you eat enough foods that contain biochemical fire extinguishers (*antioxidants*), the body is in *oxidation* or *inflammation balance*. When you eat more fire-burning foods than fire-extinguishing foods, your body suffers the wear and tear of inflammation imbalance, also known as oxidative stress.

The dial-downs don't work. Another way to understand "-itis" illnesses is to picture your body's immune-regulating system as having turn-up and turn-down dials. Normally, there is a built-in inflammation dial that turns up when the immune troops are needed and turns down when the battle is over. The reason we have an epidemic of inflammatory diseases is that the whole feverish mechanism doesn't dial down when it should. Modern diets and lifestyles, such as smoking, chronic stress, and foreign chemicals in fake food keep the inflammation dial turned up. A dial that stays turned up leads to chronic "-itises." It's like a good system within the body gone bad. Excess inflammation is now blamed as the root cause of Alzheimer's, cancer, cardiovascular disease, and just about any ailment we get. We sit too much, eat too much of the wrong things, and even think inflammatory thoughts.

To help keep the body in inflammation balance you could do three things: 1) Decrease the need for the firefighter army to come into the tissues in the first place; 2) Train the army better so that it recognizes enemies and doesn't harm civilians; 3) Be sure to eat enough fire extinguishers (antioxidants) to balance the fire starters (oxidants). That's what *The Inflammation Solution* is targeted to do.

PHARMACEUTICAL FIREFIGHTERS TO THE RESCUE

Sometimes the body's immune system, or army, needs to call in some outside reinforcements because the battle is getting out of hand. So it "buys" foreign soldiers, pharmaceutical anti-inflammatories. Of course, we have to pay these mercenaries to help fight the inflammation battle. These soldiers are trained to fight the "generic battle," but are foreign to the body. They may blunt the effects of the invasion (lessen the fire or pain), but along with that they can also damage healthy tissues. The lining of the knee joints may feel better, yet the lining of the gut (where the pharmaceutical enters) gets attacked and may even start to bleed. That's the problem with pharmaceutical soldiers. If taken too strong or too long, they not only target terrorists, but also injure civilians.

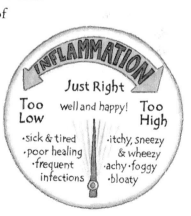

What's Your Inflammation Balance?

We doctors spend much of our time as firefighters, prescribing drugs to dampen the fires in our patients' bodies. A better solution than dispensing prescription fire extinguishers is to prevent those fires from burning out of control.

THE PROBLEM WITH PILLS

Why not just pop a pill to heal your hurts? Purchasing anti-inflammatory drugs is one of the prime reasons people visit the pharmacy. But then painful and even life-threatening, illnesses caused by anti-inflammatory drugs are one of the prime reasons people wind up in the hospital. Anti-inflammatory medications, both over-the-counter and prescription, are a good news / bad news situation. The good news is they inhibit the "bad" or "hurting" biochemicals of excess inflammation. The bad news is they also inhibit the good or healing effects of your body's natural biochemicals. And while they dial down over-inflammation in some tissues, they can dial up inflammation in other organs, such as the gut.

When your inflammatory system is dialed up too high, such as when you have arthritis, some of the biochemicals that are produced in the exaggerated inflammatory response are a group of enzymes called cyclooxygenases, or COX. The more build-up of pro-inflammatory COX chemicals (they go by scary names like *leukotrienes* and *eicosanoids*), the more the tissues, such as the lining of your knee joints, hurt. Anti-inflammatory medications lessen the production of the COX enzymes, which is why they are called "COX-inhibitors." The difference between the COX-inhibitors you buy and what your body naturally makes is like the difference between a "smart bomb" and a "dumb bomb." The COX-inhibitors that your body makes are naturally dialed to the right amount so your body heals, but it doesn't over-heal or hurt.

The "dumb bombs" of the COX-inhibitors that you buy may turn down the COX hurters in your knee joint and temporarily alleviate the arthritic pain, but they may overreact in other tissues, such as the gut and heart, causing damage to these organs. This is the problem with many pharmaceutical anti-inflammatories, and the reason some of them have been taken off the market.

Another problem with pills is they have a *rebound effect*. Remember that sometimes-annoying cytokine, histamine that you met on page 6? If you overuse antihistamines, your immune system gradually figures out that these are foreign chemicals, reacts against them, and your nose runs more than ever.

An "-itis" illness means your body is out of inflammation balance: you produce more "hurters" than "healers." While anti-inflammatory medications can inhibit the hurters, their undesirable side effects, especially intestinal upsets, mean that they top the list of worrisome medications. Not yet convinced? Google "anti-inflammatory drugs, side effects." It reads like a pathology book. For example, the many popular anti-inflammatory drugs are a real pain in the gut. The lining of your stomach produces a natural mucus layer, sort of like a protective paint that coats the sensitive lining of the stomach so that the naturally-produced acids don't eat their way through the stomach lining. The most popular medicines, called *non-steroidal anti-inflammatory drugs* (NSAIDs), can wear away some of this mucus, exposing the sensitive stomach lining to gastric juices, causing ulcers. Emergency room doctors see this scenario daily: a patient pops pills (NSAIDs), feels better, wakes up a few hours later with pain in the gut, then vomits blood and rushes to the hospital. The NSAIDs may dial down the over-inflammation in the joints (bad inflammation), but they may also suppress the normal blood-clotting regulation (good inflammation). NSAID reactions are one of the most common drug-related deaths.

There is a safer inflammation solution: the pills and skills model of *self*-care. When we get sick, we often think *pharmacologically*, "What can I *take?*" I will teach you how to first think *biologically*, "What can I *do?*"

In a later chapter you will learn about groundbreaking research on how to help your body make its own natural anti-inflammatory medicines. (To learn more about the effects of anti-inflammatory medications, read *Drug Muggers, Which Medications are Robbing Your Body of Essential Nutrients – and Natural Ways to Restore Them,* by pharmacist Suzy Cohen.)

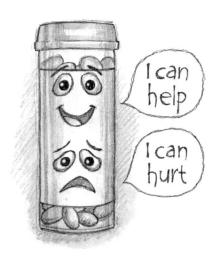

THE HORMONAL HARMONY OF HEALTH

Picture your body like a symphony orchestra. The most magnificent collection of musical artists are gathered in the most beautiful symphony hall – your body. The players in your orchestra of health are *inflammation* musicians. They actually have classical names, well, sort of: leukotrienes, eicosanoids, prostaglandins, cytokines, macrophages, interleukins, and many more. When these inflammatory hormones play in harmony, you enjoy health. When they play in disharmony, you get disease. If one section of your orchestra plays too softly, you don't heal. If one section plays too loudly, you hurt. When you keep your body in inflammation balance, beautiful music – or wellness – results. What music do you want your body to play?

Your body – the hormonal symphony of health. The instruments in a symphony orchestra are not connected to one another, so if one violin plays too loudly, the others don't automatically play softer. The hormonal symphony in your body is better. The "instruments" are wired to one another by neurochemicals called cell signalers. For example, while walking up a hill, the muscles in your lower body send signals to the heart to "pump faster, I need more blood" and to the lungs to "breathe heavier because I need more oxygen for energy." Beautiful music, or health, happens when all the instruments in your body (your hormones) tell each other how to play. That's what inflammation balance is.

YOUR BODY'S BALANCING ACT

Remember your mother preaching "eat a balanced diet"? Today Mother Scientist would add, "Keep your body in inflammation balance." Our bodies' hormonal inflammatory symphony is a beautiful balancing act of "play louder," "play softer," "get wider," "get narrower," "get more sticky," "get less sticky." These natural biochemical changes help our bodies survive and adapt to a changing environment, such as blood vessels getting wider when we run, airways getting wider when we need more air during heavy exercise, and blood getting stickier when a clot needs to form to seal a cut. Let's meet the major players in your personal symphony orchestra:

IS YOUR BODY IN BALANCE?		
Body Part/Function (Symphony Playing)	Inflammation Balance (Harmony – Wellness)	Inflammation Imbalance (Disharmony – "-itis")
Airways	Bronchodilators: need more air; Bronchoconstrictors: need less air	Allergies, asthma, wheezing

IS YOUR BODY IN BALANCE? (CONT'D)

Body Part/Function (Symphony Playing)	Inflammation Balance (Harmony – Wellness)	Inflammation Imbalance (Disharmony – "-itis")
Nasal flushing	Turn on to flush out toxins, then turn off	"Faucet" stays on, runny nose
Blood vessels	Vasodilators: need more blood; Vasoconstrictors: need less blood	High blood pressure
Heart rate	Dial up, exercise; dial down, rest	Too high, too long, heart failure
Blood clotting	Coagulants, anticoagulants	Thrombosis (clots), bleeding
Infection fighting	Pro-inflammatories and anti-inflammatories balanced; turn temperature up; turn temperature down	Infections: too many, too slow to heal, autoimmune disease
Wound healing; fighting environmental and food toxins	Play louder to heal, then play softer when healing is complete. Correctly identify "real" from "unreal" food.	Under-healing: disability; Over-healing: tissue damage, autoimmune disease

STICKY STUFF: THE ROOT CAUSE OF INFLAMMATION

My original choice for the title of this book was *Sticky Stuff*. Here is the simplest explanation of inflammation you'll ever learn. I call it my Sticky Stuff explanation of illness and aging. Let's lump all the scary-sounding inflammation biochemicals into one simple biological bag and call them "sticky stuff." Excess inflammation is the build-up of sticky stuff in your tissues, such as the amyloid deposits in the brain (Alzheimer's or cognitivitis), sticky stuff in the eyes (cataracts, macular degeneration), sticky stuff in the gums (gingivitis), sticky stuff in the walls of the blood vessels (cardiovascular disease or atherosclerosis), sticky stuff in the joints (arthritis), and sticky stuff in the skin (dermatitis). *Smooth* linings, *flexible* tissues, that's health! *Sticky* linings, *stiff* tissues, that's disease!

Returning to our concept of inflammation balance being like hormonal harmony, an orchestra inside your body having players who are mostly "smoothies" would play wellness music. An orchestra with too many "stickies" would play out of harmony, or illness music. For example, suppose a sticky player sneaks into the body's orchestra and your body experiences an unreal snack attack. Your taste buds tell you that French fry is good! Yet your internal gut police know that the French fry is not real food so they attack it. As you will learn in Chapter Two, when you put sticky stuff in your mouth, you get sticky stuff in your body. Over thousands of years the human immune system has adapted to recognize what is real and what is unreal. As the volume of unreal foods has entered the bodies of fake-food eaters, the epidemic of inflammatory diseases has skyrocketed.

The immune system army has been programmed that excess sticky stuff is not good for the body, so it attacks it. But after too many battles, too much sticky stuff builds up on the battleground, such as plaques building up on the walls of your arteries. Over the years, as sticky stuff builds up in the tissues, your immune system army may get its signals even more confused and conclude that this sticky tissue really isn't part of the body and doesn't belong there. It's a foreign invader, so it attacks it more forcefully, causing more sticky stuff. Sticky stuff! Those two memorable, child-like, but scientifically accurate words so simply describe the basis of most of the ailments that we all have at all ages. In a nutshell, *The Inflammation Solution* helps you keep sticky stuff out of your body in the first place and helps train your immune system army not to add more sticky stuff or, shall we say, not to add insult to injury. You can do that!

Sticky clumps in arteries. This is a diagram of the arteries in patients doctors treat every day. Another way to view inflammation is to imagine pro-inflammatory chemicals, such as oxidized LDL and homocysteine, as tiny sticky balls piling up on blood cells or in tissue and lumping together, especially on the lining of arteries. The immune system says, "We don't like these sticky balls so we're going to attack them (inflammatory response), which may remove some, yet leave some of these sticky balls even more sticky. Cardiologists describe the build-up of the sticky balls as "boils on the arterial walls." Imagine: when a burger and fries go into your mouth, "micro-burgers" (sticky stuff) clump onto the lining of your blood vessels. We call this "plaque."

How much sticky stuff is in your arteries?

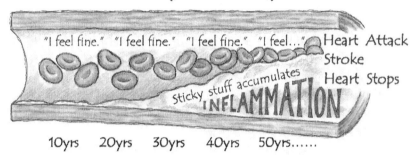

Remember "stiff" and "sticky" are the buzzwords for arterial inflammation. Stiff arterial walls lead to increased blood pressure, which lead to micro tears, which lead to more build-up of sticky stuff (plaques), leading to more high blood pressure, clots, and thrombosis. Little balls of sticky stuff break off from the arterial pavement and roll down the highway onto the off-ramp, which could result in a coronary artery clot (heart attack) or a brain artery clot (stroke).

Sticky and leaky arteries. Throughout this book you will learn about "leaky gut" and "leaky brain." Most cardiovascular disease is caused by sticky stuff damaging the arterial lining. Then sticky stuff leaks between weakened endothelial cells into the arterial walls causing hardening of the arteries. We pediatricians are now seeing cardiovascular disease, such as high blood pressure and hardening of the arteries, in ten-year-olds.

What is one of the most common medicines – and possibly one of the most harmful ones – that many people over 50 are taking? Answer: blood thinners, also called anticoagulants. Designed to reduce the level of sticky stuff – blood clotting – in arteries of the heart, brain, and other vulnerable organs, these prescription medicines can cause bleeding. Wouldn't it be safer and more effective to eat a diet that lowers sticky stuff in the blood rather than risk medicines to do it? That's exactly what our anti-inflammatory diet (see page 39) does: fewer sticky carbohydrates (carbs), fewer sticky fats, fewer sticky spikes, and therefore less build-up of sticky stuff in tissues.

To see how the modern chemical-carb diet causes sticky blood, let's go back inside one of the most fascinating surfaces in the body, the lining of your blood vessels, called the endothelium. In order to get into and nourish tissues, healthy fat and carb molecules need to worm their way from the bloodstream through channels in the endothelium and then into the tissue. But if the channels are gummed up by accumulation of sticky stuff, these nutrients can't get through. And if these molecules are chemicalized – sticky to begin with – they stick together and are too large to get through. So they are stuck inside the bloodstream, where they build up and increase blood clotting. Then it's off to the doctor to get medicines that keep the blood from over-clotting, or to the heart surgeon to ream out the sticky stuff.

My anti-sticky stuff story. In 1997, I suffered a major health crisis that birthed a series of books on healthy nutrition. Even though I "felt fine," a belated check-up revealed that my rectal bleeding was cancer. Most intestinal cancers are caused by the body's immune system at the bottom end rejecting the sticky stuff that enters the top end. I not only had major surgery, chemo and radiation therapy—I had an epiphany. As I was developing my own post-cancer-treatment health plan and upgrading my body from a state of crisis to vibrant health, I realized that even as a physician, I did not truly understand the basis of inflammation nor the causes of "-itis" illnesses. So I began to study them, and came up with the Inflammation Solution Plan. Seventeen years later I'm enjoying the two feelings of inflammation health: everything works and nothing hurts. My personal Inflammation Solution works. You'll feel the difference, too!

Over the years I have become more child-like in my writings. (Perhaps after working with children and parenting eight of them for nearly 50 years, there is an increasingly large area of my brain that thinks like a child.) That's how I came up with the sticky stuff explanation of illness and aging. I wanted a term that would, shall we say, stick. Because my readers have learned to value me as a trusted resource, it had to be accurate. "Sticky stuff" is accurate. Even my scientific friends, one a Nobel Prize winner whom you will meet on page 147, have thanked me for making science simple.

Kids get it! One of my lecture lessons is, "You put sticky stuff in your mouth, you get sticky stuff all over your body, especially in your blood vessels." A few years ago after a mother and her seven-year-old attended one of my lectures on sticky stuff, the mother told me that the following night during dinner, her child scolded her husband: "Daddy, you shouldn't put that sticky stuff in your mouth. You'll get sticky stuff in your blood." That child gave me the confidence to stick with my sticky stuff theme for this book.

Are volcanoes erupting in your arteries? Recently, while I was having lunch with Dr. John Saran, a preventive-medicine internist, John got an emergency call from one of his patients. After the call John lamented, "Another volcano eruption!" Between bites at a Mediterranean restaurant he explained that much of his day as a doctor is spent putting out volcano fires. He described the plaques (those piles of sticky stuff you just learned about) that build up in walls of blood vessels as tiny volcanoes. When the plaque gets too big, it erupts (ruptures) like a volcano and spews lava-like sticky stuff downstream to smaller vessels and tissues (think stroke, coronary thrombosis).

How doctors measure blood levels of sticky stuff. Doctors can now measure the level of your inflammation balance. (See Inflammatory Markers on page 242.) Although your doctor doesn't call the "inflammatory markers" that he or she measures "sticky stuff," that's what they are. "Markers" usually mean blood biochemicals that give a clue as to how much excess inflammation is going on in your body. One such marker that doctors frequently measure is called Hemoglobin A1c (HbA1c), also dubbed "frosted hemoglobin" (think of sugar-coated cereal), which measures the level of excess sugars that stick to the hemoglobin in your red blood cells. The higher your excess blood sugar level, the higher the HbA1c. And as you will learn on page 232, the higher the level of sticky HbA1c, the higher your chance of getting neurodegenerative diseases, such as Alzheimer's. Studies have shown that people who have a lower level of this sugary sticky stuff in their blood live healthier, longer lives and have a better inflammation balance. Remember, *The Inflammation Solution* is all about balance.

Because our body's natural ability to balance inflammation lessens as we get older, we've got to get wiser and begin following The Inflammation Solution Plan at a younger age.

An occasional bit of sticky stuff is tolerable by a young, healthy body, or at least for a short period of time. Yet, a daily dose of sticky stuff building up in tissues changes the biochemical profile of that tissue so it's no longer "self." So a smart immune system soldier says, "That's a foreigner in our system. Let's attack it." Hence the epidemic of autoimmune diseases: forms of arthritis, lupus, some forms of thyroid problems, perhaps even Alzheimer's, and some forms of diabetes. Of course, there are anti-sticky stuff prescription medicines you can buy. Yet, nature has been "prescribing" anti-sticky stuff medicines since the beginning of mankind.

THE STICKY-STUFF CYCLE OF INFLAMMATION

The three "shuns" that cause illness and aging that you will learn about in this book are:

- *Oxidation:* The body *rusts* from accumulation of sticky stuff. (More about oxidation and body rust in Chapter Two.)

- *Glycation:* Sticky stuff that accumulates in the blood and tissues when too much of the wrong food (especially sweeteners) enters the body too fast. These are appropriately called AGEs, Advanced Glycation End products, aka "sticky chemicals." Your body then gets:

- *Inflammation:* The body's wear and tear reaction to the other "shuns."

One shun triggers another. When oxidation or rust builds up (too much sticky stuff from too many fires) and glycation molecules accumulate from too much sticky food, the body perceives these "-tions" as foreign and harmful and turns up an exaggerated inflammatory response to fight them, producing more sticky stuff — excess inflammation, "-itis" illnesses. Truly a vicious cycle!

Which road are you on? Are you limping down the highway toward an "-itis" illness? The Inflammation Solution Plan will not only give your body's GPS a needed off ramp, it will take you onto the highway to health.

INFLAMMATION BALANCE MADE SIMPLE

Inflamer	Inflammation Rx
Sitting too much	Move!
Eating too much sticky stuff	Eat less sticky stuff
Thinking too many "sticky" thoughts, stress	Think more happy thoughts

That Is Easy!

Attention readers: if you are hurting so much that you want to start to heal right this minute, and wish to skip the "why it works" in each subsequent chapter, go directly to the summary of The Inflammation Solution Plan on page 266 and simply follow the checklist of what to do.

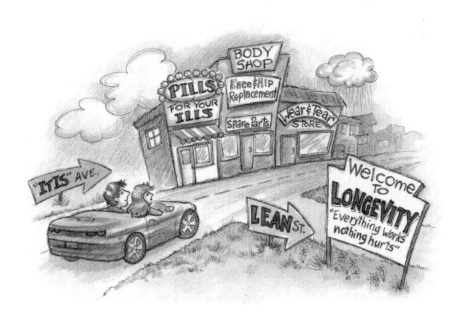

ARE YOU INFLAMMAGING?

As we age, our body's biochemistry shifts into producing more oxidants (fire starters) and less antioxidants (fire extinguishers), a deteriorating condition of stiff and sticky tissues dubbed "inflammaging." This double fault means that as we age, we must take doubly good care of ourselves. The more inflammation balance we enjoy, the younger we feel. Centenarians – people who live healthfully for a hundred years or longer 3– all seem to have a health perk in common: lower levels of excess inflammation. The top health tip for healthy aging: *keep your inflammation in balance.* As we age, so does our immune system:

- The production of some good inflammation biochemicals lessens, especially those that naturally fight infection and cancer cells.

- One of the hallmarks of inflammation balance is the body's ability to recognize self vs. non-self. As we age, the body becomes less able to always get that distinction right, so that sometimes it fights its own tissue, resulting in autoimmune diseases.

- As we age certain inflammation-producing cytokines (interferon, interleukin, and tumor necrosis factor) increase while some of the anti-inflammatory cytokines (other types of interferon) may decrease with age, further throwing the body out of balance.

- To add more insult to injury, our body's immune system becomes less selective and less protective in ridding the body of mutated cells, leaving us more prone to cancer and other "-itis" illnesses. This delayable quirk of aging is called *immunosenescence* – an old immune system. The inflammation solution keeps your immune system youthful.

- The cells and tissues of a healthy, young body are smooth and flexible. Tissues that get sick and old are stiff and sticky.

The epidemic of "-itis" illnesses – *inflammaging* – is simply due to too much sticky stuff building up in too many places too quickly throughout the body.

The polypharmacy problem. Many seniors take 8-10 pills daily. A polypharmacy is a setup for poly-problems, the so-called drug cocktail effect. Drugs are tested and FDA approved one drug at a time, not several together. Do you want to be part of an individual experiment on the unknown effects of these pills taken together?

Enjoy more mighty mitochondria. While there are many theories of why we age, one of the most accepted explanations is the *mitochondrial theory of aging*. Mitochondria are the energy batteries in the cells of your body. The more energetic a cell, the more oxidants, or sticky stuff, they produce. Younger cells produce enough natural antioxidants to quench the oxidants, thereby protecting these precious mitochondria. Like hyperactive kids, mitochondria are particularly energetic in brain, eye, and heart tissue, the three organs most likely to wear out as we age. Two mitochondrial dysfunctions (sorry, another "dysfunction") can occur as we age:

1. Aging mitochondria produce more oxidants, or more sticky stuff. The main culprits are called superoxide and hydrogen peroxide.

2. Aging mitochondria produce less antioxidants to quench the fire of the excess oxidants.

Like big words? One of the fire-quenching antioxidants is called *superoxide dismutase*. Translation: I keep this wild kid from getting out of control.

The mitochondrial dysfunction of aging can be delayed by what Mom always said: "Eat more fruits, vegetables, and seafood and go outside and play." In scientific mother lingo, "Eat more antioxidants and move your body to make more antioxidants." To take this maternal advice one step further: "The longer we age, the more antioxidants we need to eat and the more we need to move."

ENJOY THE ANTI-INFLAMMATORY EFFECTS OF ANTIOXIDANTS

Before you learn the list of anti-inflammatory foods in the next chapter, you need to understand the powerful nutrients in these foods that make them so anti-inflammatory – the other A-word – antioxidants. When it comes to healing inflamed body parts, doctors preach: *The tissue is the issue.* Simply put, the less sticky stuff that gets into tissues, the less they get damaged by inflammation. While the root cause of most illnesses and aging is inflammation, the root cause of most inflammation is another "shun" – *oxidation*. Like inflammation, oxidation balance is healing. Oxidation imbalance is hurting. Like your car engine produces exhaust from burning fuel, your body's engine, its metabolism, produces exhaust we call *oxidants* or by-products of normal oxygen burning. Oxidation is a good thing to fuel healthy tissues. In fact, oxidants (also called free radicals) may act like microscopic antibiotics to attack germs that get into the cells. Yet, the *excess* production of oxidants, *oxidative stress,* damages tissues and invokes an exaggerated inflammatory response that adds more tissue damage, or inflames the tissues. What happens with excess oxidation in the body is like what happens when the oxygen in the air reacts with unprotected metal – it rusts. While it doesn't sound so sexy, when we age too fast or get sick too often, we rust. Another way to understand the aging process: *inflammaging is rusting. The Inflammation Solution* is an anti-rust program.

EASING AGING	
Inflammation Problem	**Inflammation Solution**
We "rust" (oxidation) (page 26).	Eat an anti-inflammatory diet (page 39).
Joints stiffen.	Move more! (page 145).
Tissue repair slows.	Do more of the above two solutions.
Immune system weakens.	Do an immune-support L.E.A.N. (Lifestyle, Exercise, Attitude, Nutrition) Program (page 34).
We produce more AGEs (page 45) in tissues, especially in joints, brain, skin, and gut.	Eat a less AGE-producing diet (page 39).
Digestion slows, heartburn happens.	Graze; the smaller the meal, the better you'll feel. Enjoy the sipping solution (page 57).
Blood sugar regulation gets more challenging.	Eat a blood-sugar-stabilizing diet (page 39).
Falls are more likely.	Do more balance exercises.
We lose muscle mass.	Do more strength-building exercises.
Vision lessens.	Eat more seafood (page 46).
Medications have more undesirable side effects.	Practice the pills-and-skills model of self-care, with your first emphasis on skills (page 13).
Sleep is more interrupted.	Enjoy sleep-well strategies (page 184).
Brain is less able to handle stress.	Learn stressbusters (page 180).
Metabolism slows.	Eat less quantity, better quality (page 124).
Height shrinks, waist expands.	Do all of the above, so that waist shrinks and height stays the same.

My friend, Paula Bickford, Ph.D, a neuroscientist at the University of South Florida - Center of Excellence for Aging and Brain Repair, uses the Tin Man in *The Wizard of Oz* as an example of oxidation of the brain. Oxidation caused the Tin Man to rust until Dorothy came along and oiled him. You will learn which antioxidant oils in food help prevent our brains from rusting.

Enter antioxidants. Since the body naturally produces oxidants, or wear-and-tear chemicals, it would seem logical that the body would need to consume *antioxidants* to keep it in balance, and that's just what Dr. Mother Nature prescribes. When the cells in your body burn food for energy, they burn oxygen as well. When oxygen is burned, exhaust molecules called "free radicals" are released. Excess free radicals are like vandals loose in your body. They have at least one extra electron, giving them a negative charge, which drives them around the body looking for cells with which they can react. These reactions damage the DNA and other substances in cells. Much of the time the cells can

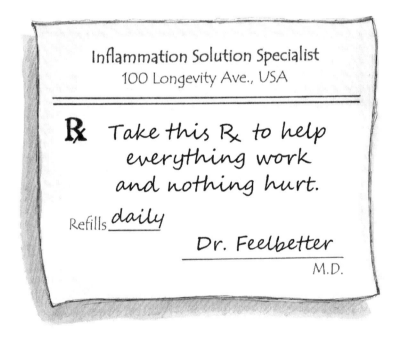

Inflammation Solution Specialist
100 Longevity Ave., USA

℞ Take this ℞ to help everything work and nothing hurt.

Refills *daily*

Dr. Feelbetter
M.D.

repair themselves, but the cell neighborhood can't protect itself from these gangs of free radicals all by itself.

Enter the antioxidant "police." Antioxidant molecules have a positive charge, so when they meet up with negatively charged free radicals, they neutralize, or "handcuff", them so they can't do any damage. Your body needs more antioxidant police officers as you get older, since the body's ability to repair itself diminishes with age. Antioxidants also help to prevent damage by carcinogens, such as ultraviolet radiation, tobacco smoke, and environmental pollutants.

THE THREE BIG As

These are the top antioxidants for The Inflammation Solution:

- Astaxanthin, the pink antioxidant in seafood (page 87)
- Colorful fruits and vegetables
- Omega-3 fish oils

Doctor's orders: eat more fruits and vegetables and go fish!

One of the reasons mothers preach, "Eat more fruits, vegetables and seafood" is that the nutrients that make these foods so colorful – and so healthful – are antioxidants. For example, the red pigment in a tomato is the antioxidant lycopene that protects the plant from sunburn. These colorful "Nature's medicines" go by biochemical-sounding names such as: carotenoids (the yellow, orange, and red pigments in fruits and vegetables, and the pink pigment in seafood), flavonoids (found in grape skins), isoflavones (found in legumes and soy products), and anthocyanins (the antioxidant that makes blueberries blue). And it's not only plants that produce antioxidants.

Seafood, such as wild salmon, produces the powerful antioxidant astaxanthin to protect their tissues during their marathon swim upstream.

Back to our army analogy. Antioxidants are like the mechanics and garbage collectors that keep the military camp and its equipment clean and working. Antioxidants clean up the mess of the battlefield left by the army, scrub rust off the equipment, and carry away waste products. I formulated and follow my six-S anti-inflammatory diet (see next chapter) mainly because it is so high in antioxidants. In myself and in my patients I notice the antioxidant effect mainly in five organs. Antioxidants help your:

- *eyes* see better
- *brain* think clearer
- *heart* pump stronger
- *joints* work easier
- *skin* look younger and feel smoother

The delicate dance. To keep yourself in inflammation balance, your body is doing a continual delicate dance between the *oxidants* we produce during normal metabolism and the *antioxidants* we make and eat to keep this dance going in a healthful direction.

In summary, you can control your inflammation by:

1. Producing fewer fires (oxidants)

2. Making more fire extinguishers (antioxidants)

3. Both: this is The Inflammation Solution

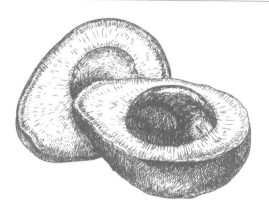

THE CASE OF THE "INFLAMED" AVOCADO

Try this experiment. Halve an avocado. Pour lemon juice (an antioxidant, anti-inflammatory) on one half. In around six hours you will notice the unprotected half is obviously "inflamed" or oxidized. It looks withered, sick and old. Which avocado half do you want your body to be like?

PART II

THE INFLAMMATION SOLUTION

Imagine having a body where everything works and nothing hurts – the two goals of good health. You will now learn the tools to help you achieve these goals. In Part I, you learned that the main inflammation problem is accumulating too much sticky stuff in your vital organs. In Part II you will learn:

- How to keep sticky stuff from entering your body in the first place.
- How to keep sticky stuff from accumulating in your tissues if some gets into your body.
- How to make your own natural anti-inflammatory medicines to clean up the sticky stuff before it damages the tissues and you get an "-itis".

Our Inflammation Solution Plan to heal your hurts is summarized by the acronym L.E.A.N.:

How you *live:*	Lifestyle
How you *move:*	Exercise
How you *think*:	Attitude
How you *eat*:	Nutrition

CHAPTER 2

Eat the Anti-inflammatory Diet

Yes, food can heal your hurts. Remember our simple explanation of inflammation: sticky stuff accumulates throughout your body (especially in the brain, eyes, heart, joints, skin, and gut – all those "-itis" areas). Let's now expand our sticky stuff explanation to: when you put sticky-stuff-producing food in your mouth, you get sticky-stuff accumulating in your body. What goes into your mouth is the top cause – and can be the top healer – of excess inflammation. Changing what goes into your mouth is the easiest change to make that produces the quickest results.

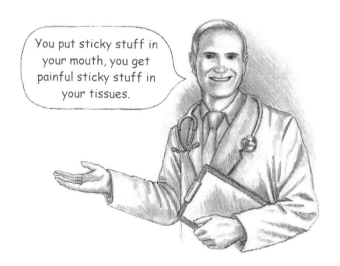

You put sticky stuff in your mouth, you get painful sticky stuff in your tissues.

FOUR REASONS WHY FAST FOOD IS SO INFLAMMATORY

Once upon a time people ate real food. We had fewer sticky-stuff spikes and fewer inflammatory illnesses. Over the past few decades, the more that food became fake the more our bodies got sore. Here's why.

The Food Inflammation Problem

1. Foods lose their "wholeness." When we eat "whole foods", the body takes them in with a welcoming immune response. We are taking in all the fiber, fat, and protein that nature puts there and we naturally avoid hormone spikes in our blood after eating. To make food cheaper to produce and longer-lasting on a shelf, though, vital elements are removed, for example, the germ and bran from wheat. The processed foods that enter the delivery trucks have become "fake" and "fast" by having over 50 percent of their wholeness, the very nutrients that keep us healthy, replaced with chemicals. When we eat these foods, the body's immune system gets confused and greets them with an unnatural and unhealthy response: we get sticky-stuff spikes and become inflamed.

2. Foods lose their balance. Real foods (such as free-range animals eating grass) have the right balance of fats, especially the right ratio of omega-3 to omega-6 fats: around 1:1 to 1:2. Feeding livestock grains instead of grass causes an omega imbalance, and helps put the animal in inflammation imbalance. When real foods get diverted to food factories, more omega-6s are put in (they're cheaper and last longer on the shelf) and more omega-3s are taken out (they're more expensive and spoil faster). As a result, our modern diet suffers from a ratio of between 1:10 and 1:20 of omega-3 (anti-inflammatory) to omega-6 (pro-inflammatory) oils. This downgrading of fats in foods is thought to be one of the prime contributors to the epidemic of inflammatory illnesses.

3. Foods lose their natural sweetness. Once upon a time, real foods provided low after-eating sugar spikes, or what is now termed a "low glycemic load." Again, that's because the protein, fiber, and fat in real foods slow down the sugar rush. When food chemists realized that the sugar component of food is the cheapest and that the sweet taste stimulates overeating, natural foods became refined and we were left with sugary sticky stuff, and even artificial sweetness (think frosted cereals, sweetened beverages, and so on). This has led to a huge increase in the inflammatory illnesses of insulin-resistance, or type 2 diabetes, and one of the most serious and debilitating of autoimmune diseases, type I diabetes.

4. Foods lose their medicinal effects. For millennia, food was known as medicine. In the last few decades, though, not only have the medicinal qualities been taken out of the foods we eat, but those fake foods cause us to need more store-bought medicines. The greatest medicinal loss has been in antioxidants, the colorful plant nutrients, or "phytonutrients," that are responsible for food being known as "nature's medicine" and are the reason behind Dr. Mom's medicinal advice to "put more color on your plate." The side trip through the food factory de-colored our diet (think white bread and white pasta) and Americans got fatter and more inflamed.

THE FOOD INFLAMMATION SOLUTION

Those are the four main food causes of the inflammation problem. Naturally, the four solutions are:

    1. Eat whole foods.

2. Eat foods with a healthy omega balance.

3. Eat foods with a sugar balance, sugars naturally partnered with spike-less nutrients (healthy fats, protein, and fiber).

4. Eat foods rich in antioxidants – put more color on your plate.

These are the features of the anti-inflammatory diet you will soon learn to enjoy.

Top inflammation solution: Eat less sticky stuff.

If you wonder why around 70 percent of The Inflammation Solution involves food choices, that's because 70 percent of the problem is what and how we eat, and 70 percent of the immune system resides in the gut. You will now learn which foods are pro-inflammatory (promote inflammation imbalance) and which foods are anti-inflammatory (promote inflammation balance).

Fix your gut first. When you relieve the "-itis" in your intestines, you're likely to also lessen the "-itises" throughout the rest of your body.

Foods that promote inflammation balance have one or more of three effects:

1. They contain less sticky stuff and therefore deposit less sticky stuff in your tissues.

2. They feed the inflammation army the right nutrients to promote a healthy balance between pro-inflammatory and anti-inflammatory reactions in the body.

3. They lessen biochemical reactions within the body that promote the deposition of sticky stuff on tissues, namely oxidation and glycation, described on page 22.

DR. BILL'S "SIX-S" ANTI-INFLAMMATORY DIET

Following my own life-threatening "-itis" illness, I thoroughly researched what diet would best balance my inflammation. After a few years of experimentation – and taste-reshaping – I came up with a simple, delicious and nutritious diet. We'll call it the six-S diet. ("Diet" simply means a way of eating. We're all on a "diet.") Instead of a diet, call it a "do-it."

1. Seafood: primarily wild pacific salmon.

2. Smoothies: multiple dark-colored fruits, berries, organic yogurt, ground flaxseeds, and more. The *sipping solution* is one of the best inflammation solutions. (See Sipping Solution, page 57).

3. Salads: go as deeply colorful as you can. Go green, such as organic arugula, kale and spinach; go red, such as tomatoes and red peppers; add red or black beans.

4. Spices: turmeric, black pepper, ginger, garlic, rosemary, chilis, and cinnamon

5. Satisfying snacks: graze to your body's content. (See why grazing is good for you, page 119)

6. Supplements: The three inflammation-balancing ones I use in my medical practice and those supported by science:

   - Omega-3 fish oils, primarily salmon oil from Alaska

   - Astaxanthin, the natural anti-inflammatory nutrient that makes salmon pink. We recommend Hawaiian astaxanthin.

   - Juice Plus+®, a whole-food-based concentrate of many fruits and vegetables

DR. BILL'S "SIX-S" ANTI-INFLAMMATORY DIET *(CONT'D)*

These science-based supplements are meant to fill in the gaps in the first three S's: seafood, salads, and smoothies, since few people consistently eat an average of two ounces of wild salmon every day and ten servings (ten fistfuls) of combined fruits and vegetables every day. (On page 83, we'll discuss each of these supplements in scientific detail.) For more about these supplements, see:

- The Omega-3 Effect: Everything You Need to Know About the Supernutrient for Living Longer, Happier, and Healthier (Sears and Sears, Little Brown 2012)

- Natural Astaxanthin – Hawaii's Supernutrient, by William Sears, M.D. 2015

- AskDrSears.com/JuicePlusResearch

Think of the "savory six" as the peacekeepers in the inflammation war going on in your body. They quench the fires of inflamma*tion*, blunt the sugar spikes of glyca*tion*, and soften the wear and tear of oxida*tion*. Remember, for good health, keep the excess "shuns" out of your body.

THE SAD DIET VS. THE SIX-S INFLAMMATION-BALANCING DIET

The Standard American Diet (SAD) produces "-itis" illnesses because it has the double whammy of being heavy in oxidants (wear-and-tear biochemicals) and lower in antioxidants (repair biochemicals). This imbalance between too high of wear-and-tear chemicals and too low of repair chemicals leads to immune imbalance, or illness. Notice in the previous illustration that when you eat primarily the six-S diet, a healthy amount of oxidants are produced to give you the energy you need. Smart Dr. Mother Nature provides lots of antioxidants in these

Is Your Body in Balance?

What's your sticky stuff level?

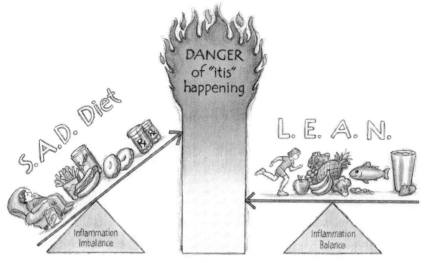

INFLAMETER

Sticky stuff level in blood

foods to balance your normal metabolism. This results in inflammation balance and wellness.

Once you stop the SAD, your body will feel these anti-inflammatory effects of the six-S diet:

You will feel more satisfied with less food. Because these foods have a *high nutrient density* (more nutrients per calorie), you will automatically eat less, the consequences of which are:

- Less food being metabolized means less sticky stuff (oxidation) being produced in your body. Less oxidants and more antioxidants is a recipe for longevity. (See page 143 for why eating less lessens inflammation.)

- A leaner waist results in less wear-and-tear inflammatory chemicals being released into your blood and tissues. (See page 163 to learn how a leaner waist lessens inflammation.)

You will crave real foods. You will gradually reshape your tastes as you progress from: "Don't like but must eat to feel better" – to "like" – to "crave." Once you reach the crave stage, it will feel like you turned on some internal switch that continually prompts you, "Keep eating this way. It's good for you."

We are what we absorb. Over centuries, both the nutrient nature of food and the lining of our intestines adapted to welcome each other. If your gut could talk it would say, "We welcome real food for real gut health." This is why the gut typically absorbs a higher percentage of real foods from nature than it does the synthetic foods from a food factory. Like a protective mother, the gut is a picky eater, as if to say, "This is real food, so I'll let more of it into my body." Or, if a fake food enters it may shout, sometimes painfully, "You don't belong here, so I'll reject most of you!" And that "rejection" comes in the form of a painful and often debilitating "-itis" of the intestines, inflammatory bowel disease.

The real food diet. If someone inquires, "What is the anti-inflammatory diet?" simply respond, "It's a real food diet."

Less of a load. When deciding to eat a certain food, I often consider, "How much of an inflammatory load does this meal have?" Real foods, like our ancestral diet (known as the "paleo" diet) naturally have a low inflammatory load.

AVOID SPIKES

The six-S anti-inflammatory diet avoids spikes. Before we go through each one of these S's, showing you how eating more of them can help you feel your own anti-inflammatory effect, I want you to understand the top S-word for inflammation health: *spikes*. The simplest way to summarize the anti-inflammatory diet: *avoid sticky spikes*. Spikes is the bad word for inflammation. If your blood could talk, it would plead, "No sticky-stuff spikes, please!" It is the buzzword doctors use to describe sudden high levels of sticky stuff in your blood, often from the sticky stuff food chemists spike food with. The medical terms for foods and drinks that spike are: *postprandial lipemia* (after eating you get fatty spikes in the blood) and *postprandial glycemia* (after eating you get sugary spikes in the blood). The term for foods and drinks that spike less is *lipemia/glycemia blunting*. Let's see what happens in your body and blood when you get spikes.

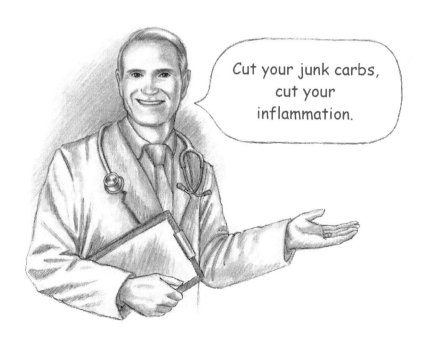

Cut your junk carbs, cut your inflammation.

While writing this section, I consulted my friend, Dr. Vince Fortanasce, Professor of Neurology at the University of Southern California School of Medicine and author of *The Anti-Alzheimer's Prescription*. Dr. Vince liked my "spikes" and "sticky stuff" explanation of Alzheimer's disease. He explained that high fructose corn syrup causes higher insulin spikes than cane sugar, allowing more amyloid (sticky stuff) to be deposited in brain tissue.

The biochemical process that goes on in the bloodstream after a meal is like rush-hour traffic on a highway. Imagine those annoying, but safe, stoplights on freeway on-ramps. They turn on during rush-hour to keep too many cars from entering the freeway too fast and clogging traffic. If only we could enjoy such an internal traffic controller when we eat. It would prompt us to slow down the food entering the digestive highway to allow sufficient time to move the food along from the mouth to its place of employment, the tissues,

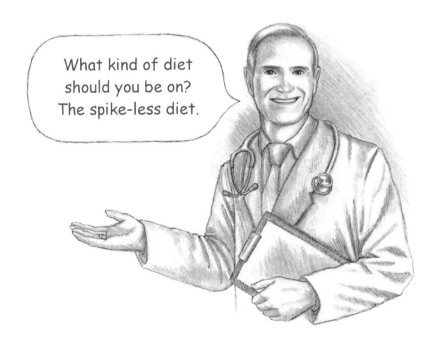

without getting piled up along the roadside (stuck in the gut or deposited on the lining of your blood vessels).

THREE TIPS TO SPIKE-LESS DINING

- Eat a large salad at beginning of meal (page 127)
- Graze to the rule of twos (page 117)
- Eat spike-less foods (page 126)

The opposite of "spikes" is "slow" and "stable." As you've already learned, the more stable your blood chemistry, the more stable your inflammation balance. Big meals are bad for the body. When too much food goes into your gut and into your bloodstream too quickly, the body signals "overload," "traffic congestion," and your inflammation police muster up the immune system to clean up the mess. Excess food puts your body into a hypermetabolic state of oxidative stress called *food energy toxicity*. When you eat too much food too fast, not only is your stomach bloated, you also bloat your bloodstream by overloading it with excess sticky sugars and fat. Your body tries to quickly burn the excess food, which generates more internal micro fires, resulting in exaggerated inflammation, or oxidative stress. These micro fires are also known as accelerated glycation end products (AGEs) or sticky sugars. To add more inflammatory insult to inflammatory injury, your body pours out more insulin (excess insulin causes excess inflammation) to store the excess food as fat (usually around the waist). Since the body does not like to "waste food", it "waists" food. (See related sections: Graze, page 117; Toxic Waist, page 164; and A Tale of Two Fuels, page 114.)

Now let's learn how each of the six-S foods helps balance your inflammation.

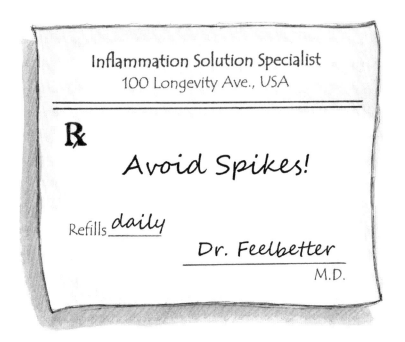

Inflammation Solution Specialist
100 Longevity Ave., USA

℞

Avoid Spikes!

Refills *daily*

Dr. Feelbetter

M.D.

SEAFOOD

People who eat the most seafood tend to live the longest and hurt the least. Seafood is the top inflammation balancer for *all organs* at *all ages*.

Three top inflammation-balancing nutrients are found in pink seafood: Omega-3 oils, vitamin D, and the pink powerhouse astaxanthin, which you will learn about on page 87. The two omega-3 fats in fish oil, DHA and EPA, are some of Dr. Mother Nature's top anti-inflammatory nutrients. As you learned on page 9, a healthful inflammation balance is when the *healers* (your immune system soldiers that clean up after the battle) balance the *inflamers* (those soldiers that fought the battle and killed the germs in the first place). Omega-3s help keep your immune system from overproducing too many fighters in addition to helping your body release more healers. In a nutshell,

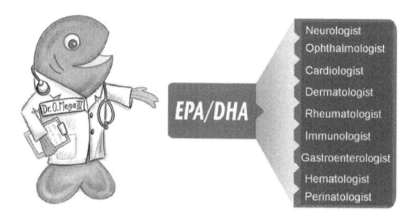

omega-3 fish oils tame the excess biochemical inflamers that circulate through your body causing the "-itis" illnesses. Let's go deeper into the "-itis" areas of your body and see how these oily anti-inflammatories work.

For healthy inflammation balance, go fish! A time-tested medical truism is: Your body is only as healthy as each cell in it. Each cell is surrounded by a flexible sac called the cell membrane, most of which is fat. The healthier the fat in the sac, the healthier the cell membrane. One of the top fats in the cell membrane is the omega-3 fat found in fish oil. A healthy cell membrane has just the right permeability to let in the right balance of inflammation biochemicals – not so much as to damage the vulnerable cell membrane, but just enough to keep it healthy. So far you have learned that inflammation that makes the body sore is caused by overproduction of biochemical byproducts – let's call them "hurters" – that outnumber the "healers." The omega-3 fats in fish oils are healers. Imagine the omega-3 fats in fish oil "swimming" into all the cells of your body and balancing inflammation by putting out the fires or extinguishing the overproduction of tissue inflamers (biochemically called "inflammatory eicosanoids").

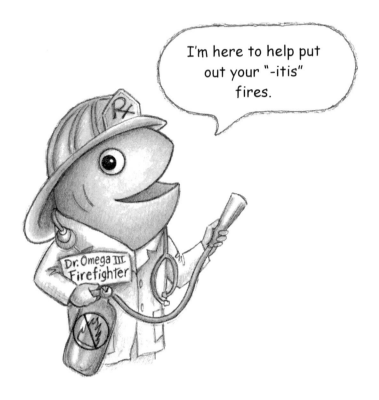

My anti-inflammatory fish story. In 2006, I had the privilege of fishing for a week in Norway with Dr. Jorn Dyerberg, the acknowledged father of omega-3 fish-oil science. In 2011, I had the privilege of hosting him for a roundtable discussion on omega-3 science updates. He loved my sticky-stuff explanation of inflammatory illnesses. I asked him, "What was your first clue that seafood was an anti-inflammatory or anti-sticky-stuff food?" He related that in the early seventies, during the height of the "fat is bad" craze, the blood tests he performed revealed that people who ate more seafood (a high-fat but a right-fat diet) had lower levels of sticky stuff (factors that made the blood clot too quickly) and a healthier inflammation balance than people who ate less seafood. Thirty years and over 22,000 journal articles later, the fish-reduces-sticky-stuff hypothesis has been proven true.

Science Says: Go Fish!

Here's a summary of what science says about the inflammation-balancing effects of omega-3 fish oils*.

Brain

- Improves learning and behavior in kids
- Mellows moods
- Prevents Alzheimer's
- Improves thinking
- Helps heal neurodegenerative diseases
- Lessens stroke

Ears

- Delays age-related hearing loss

Eyes

- Improves vision
- Moistens dry eyes
- Delays age-related macular degeneration

Gums

- Helps gingivitis

Gut

- Lessens colitis and irritable bowel syndrome

Immune System

- Lessens autoimmune diseases

Heart

- Steadies irregular heartbeat
- Lessens clots in vessels
- Balances high blood pressure
- Softens atherosclerosis

Lungs

- Alleviates asthma and bronchitis

Skin

- Heals dermatitis

Joints

- Alleviates arthritis

Penis

- Enhances blood vessel health for erectile function

See related section: Give yourself an oil change, page 141.

*For more helpful information on how omega-3s help heal all the "-itis" illnesses, see *The Omega-3 Effect*, Little Brown, 2012.

As you can see, omega-3s help balance inflammation in all organs, yet their most healthful effects are in the heart and brain.

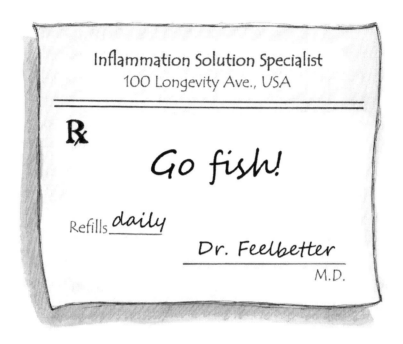

How omega-3s help heal the heart. Most cardiovascular diseases are caused by the build-up of sticky stuff on the lining of the blood vessels, called the endothelium. Here's how most cardiovascular disease develops:

- Sticky stuff gets into the blood and invades the lining of the blood vessels, the endothelium, causing a rough surface.
- Sticky stuff collects on the surface of the blood cells causing them to stick together, slowing blood flow, causing clots: stroke, coronary thrombosis.
- The inflammatory system, like a core of reactive highway engineers, floats into the blood vessels to repair a damaged surface. Sometimes they overreact and over repair, leading to

the build-up of more plaque, more sticky stuff, and more inflammation, resulting in atherosclerosis. Instead of your blood vessels being smooth and flexible, they become stiff and sticky, leading to high blood pressure.

Omega-3s act as both anti-inflammatories and anti-coagulants to tame the road crew from overreacting and lessen the build-up and the break-offs of plaque, which eventually clog the vessels. In heart doctor talk - sticky stuff in the blood leads to stiff arteries. The main anti-inflammatory effect of omega-3s is to lessen the build-up of sticky stuff inside the arteries. Per the medical truism, "Your tissues are only as healthy as the blood vessels supplying them," much of the inflammation-balancing effects of omega-3 fish oils on all organs are due to the healthier vessels. (See more on endothelial health, page 152).

Notice how omega-3 fish oils get into red blood cell membranes, keeping red blood cells from sticking together and forming clots in blood vessels. And omega-3s help keep sticky stuff inflammation off the lining of the blood vessels. The following passage is from *The Omega-3 Effect* (Little Brown 2012):

- Cardiovascular disease is now considered primarily an inflammation issue rather than just a cholesterol problem. Statins may have their healing effect as an anti-inflammatory medicine more than as a cholesterol-lowering drug. A famous study that helped turn the tide from the cholesterol theory of cardiovascular disease to excess inflammation as the root cause was the JUPITER Heart Study – researchers found that statins not only lowered LDL cholesterol, but also lowered the inflammation marker CRP (c-reactive protein) and thus lowered heart disease.

Cardiologists conclude that omega-3s make blood flow to tissues more fluid. There are even names for the anti-inflammatories that are increased by eating more omega-3s, such as *protectins* and *resolvins*. In summary, one of the best ways to soften your tissues, increase blood flow to tissues, and help them be healthier and last longer is to go fish! (See Cognitivitis, page 230, on how to reduce inflammation of the brain.)

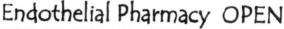

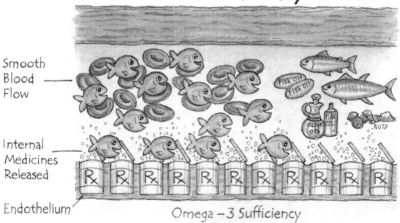

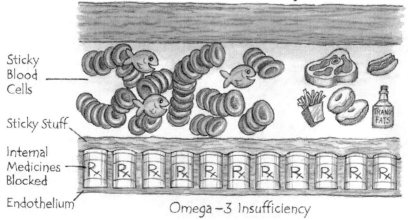

OMEGA BALANCE HELPS INFLAMMATION BALANCE

Once upon a time when humans ate from the land and sea instead of from the bottle and box, their blood was less sticky, presumably because they ate less sticky fats and sugars. Then our bodies got an "oil change". Humans began eating more factory-processed oils and less seafood oils.

Science confirms that people who eat too much omega-6 oils and too little omega-3 oils have more sticky stuff in their blood. Specifically, their blood cells stick together more. Recent research concludes that persons who have a better omega balance (eating more omega-3s and less omega-6 oils) show less sticky stuff in their blood, less sticky stuff in their tissues, less sticky stuff on their cell membranes, and less inflammatory markers (the measurements of sticky stuff levels in your blood).

Omega-3s get inside your genes. For those of you who want a second helping of how this works at the genetic level, let's go inside your genes. The latest buzzword in health is *epigenetics*, meaning how genes turn up or turn down their expression of biochemical language for health or illness. Sufficient omega-3s are especially vital to children with genetic differences. Our son, Stephen, has Down syndrome. We can't change his genes, but we can influence how they are expressed. One of his favorite slogans is "Go fish!" As you learned on page 10, think of your genes that regulate your inflammation balance as having dials, those to dial up your inflammation system when you need it, say to fight infection, and genes to dial down the levels of inflammatory biochemicals when you need less of them, so you don't get an "-itis". Omega-3s regulate the dial on the genes so they express themselves more healthfully, neither turning up too high or too low. A body in this state is in balance at the genetic level.

Think of inflammation imbalance as your body's police and infection-fighters being on hyper alert, sort of an inflammatory anxiety disorder. Omega-3s know all the moves of these hyperactive cells, so they can put the body's defense system back in balance.

GO WILD! BE LESS INFLAMED

My top anti-inflammatory food pick is *Wild Pacific Sockeye salmon*, mainly because of the synergistic effects of the omega-3 oils and astaxanthin, the antioxidant powerhouse that makes wild salmon pink. Both omega-3s and astaxanthin are together in their natural form in wild salmon, unlike farmed Atlantic salmon, which are fed synthetic astaxanthin from petrochemicals to color the flesh. (See more about natural Hawaiian astaxanthin, page 87.)

Cardiologist Dr. Mark Houston, Professor of Medicine at Vanderbilt University, makes the point that eating *wild*, not farmed fish, is the best way to promote inflammation balance. His research reveals that once fish farms started feeding their fish a sticky-stuff diet (more grains and less seafood), the fish flesh we eat changed to more pro-inflammatory fats and less anti-inflammatory fats – just like what happens to our bodies when we eat out of the food factory. We went from being "wild humans" enjoying inflammation balance to being factory-fed humans suffering from inflammation imbalance. If you must eat farmed fish, enjoy salmon and trout, not tilapia and catfish (two highly farmed fish that are way out of omega balance – having too-high levels of omega-6s and much lower levels of omega-3s than other fish). Fish and meats that have a high ratio of omega-6s-to-omega-3s are called "foods with high inflammatory potential."

Because of the highly researched lipid-lowering effect of omega-3s, many cardiologists recommend that high doses of omega-3s (two to four grams per day of DHA and EPA combined) be the first line of treatment in reducing triglyceride and sticky cholesterol levels. Certainly, if statin drugs are needed, cardiologists recommend that they be used in addition to, but not instead of, omega-3 fish oils.

CHOOSE SEAFOODS HIGHEST IN ANTI-INFLAMMATORY OMEGA-3 OILS

- *Best choice:* wild Pacific salmon. Eating 12 ounces per week gives you around *600 mg* EPA/DHA per day, depending on the species. (See omega-3 supplement doses, page 84.)
- *Good choices:* anchovies, sardines, tuna
- *Don't eat:* swordfish, shark or marlin. Many farmed fish, especially tilapia and catfish, are not only low in omega-3 EPA/DHA, but are high in omega-6s, leading to inflammation imbalance. We discourage eating these fish if you have an "-itis" illness.

Dr. Bill recommends: "VitalChoice.com is my favorite online *pharma-sea.*"

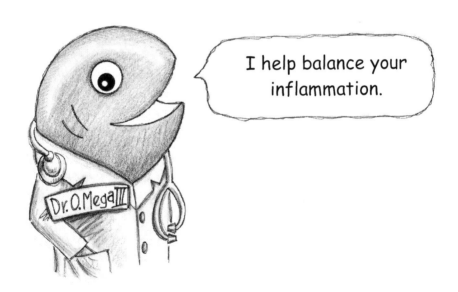

I help balance your inflammation.

For more details about safe and omega-3 rich seafood and the content of omega-3 EPA/DHA in various seafood, see DrSearsWellnessInstitute.org/resources/inflammation/safeseafood and Resources page 267.

SMOOTHIES: ENJOY THE SIPPING SOLUTION

The sipping solution is a major part of The Inflammation Solution. This supergrazing way of eating can put your body into inflammation balance quickly and easily.

My smoothie story. To put my own body into biochemical balance following my health crisis in 1997, I realized that grazing was the way to go. Being impatient, I wanted to see and feel the fastest results. That's how I came up with the sipping solution for inflammation balance. I've continued this way of eating and advise it to many of the inflamed patients in my medical practice. I believe it is the simplest and one of the smartest changes that you can make, and it will allow you to see and feel the quickest results. Let's get started.

Start low, go slow. Any time you make a big change in the way you eat, your gut brain may get a bit nervous since the body, especially the gut, doesn't like sudden, drastic changes. So ease into this new way of eating. Begin with once a week, twice a week, and so on as your gut tells you. Start with a few of the listed ingredients that you most need and most like and gradually add more of the inflammation-balancing foods as your perseverance and gut voice tells you. Be sure to begin by sipping a smaller amount slowly, and gradually increasing the volume, until you're slowly drinking a blender-full throughout the day. Four to five days a week, I begin my day in inflammation balance by making a smoothie full of anti-inflammatory foods, rich in antioxidants, rich in satisfying and blood-insulin-stabilizing nutrients, and I sip on it all day long. It's my breakfast, lunch, and snacks. Then I enjoy a nutritious dinner. See my personal recipe on page 61. Which recipe is for you? The one you will do!

DR. BILL'S SMOOTHIE PRESCRIPTION

- Select choices from each of the five food categories below. Begin with the ingredients that you already know you like.
- Be sure to add *protein* and *healthy fats* to each smoothie, which will taste better and keep you fuller longer than a carb-only smoothie. Our basic recipes are 20-25 percent protein, 20-25 percent fats, and 50 percent carbs.
- Begin with one 12-ounce smoothie at breakfast, two to three days a week.
- Gradually increase to a breakfast smoothie a day, five days a week.
- Gradually increase the volume of the smoothie you make from 12 ounces (one glass) to as much as 64 ounces, or five glasses (the volume of most blenders such as the Vitamix).

Healthy Fluids

- Coconut milk/coconut water
- Almond milk
- Goat milk
- Green tea
- Organic juices: green, carrot, vegetable, pomegranate

Healthy Proteins

- Organic Greek yogurt
- Nut butters
- Hawaiian spirulina
- Chocolate or vanilla healthy protein powder, multi-nutrient mix (I like Juice Plus+ Complete®)

Healthy Fats

- Avocado
- Nut butters
- Ground flaxseeds or chia seeds
- Coconut oil, virgin

Healthy Carbs

- Blueberries
- Strawberries
- Pomegranates
- Papaya
- Kiwi
- Banana
- Greens
- Kale
- Spinach
- Chard

Special additions

- Cinnamon

- Wheat germ
- Hawaiian spirulina
- Cacao
- Figs/raisins/dates
- Shredded coconut
- Grated ginger
- Mint

Now you're ready to feel the full health benefits of the sipping solution. Sip on your 64-ounce smoothie in frequent mini-meals throughout the day: it's your breakfast, lunch, mid-morning and mid-afternoon snack. Then eat a healthy dinner.

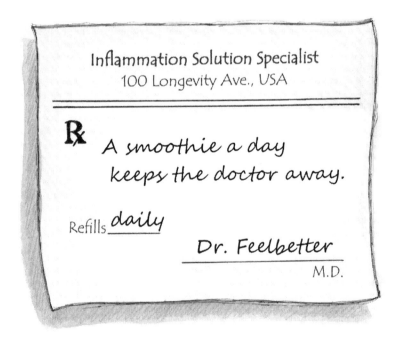

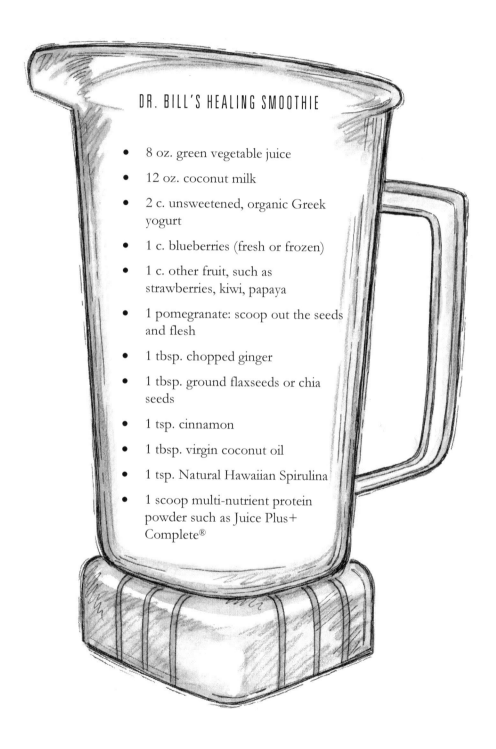

DR. BILL'S HEALING SMOOTHIE

- 8 oz. green vegetable juice

- 12 oz. coconut milk

- 2 c. unsweetened, organic Greek yogurt

- 1 c. blueberries (fresh or frozen)

- 1 c. other fruit, such as strawberries, kiwi, papaya

- 1 pomegranate: scoop out the seeds and flesh

- 1 tbsp. chopped ginger

- 1 tbsp. ground flaxseeds or chia seeds

- 1 tsp. cinnamon

- 1 tbsp. virgin coconut oil

- 1 tsp. Natural Hawaiian Spirulina

- 1 scoop multi-nutrient protein powder such as Juice Plus+ Complete®

DR. BILL'S HEALING SMOOTHIE (*CONT'D*)

Special additions for taste and satiety:

- 1 tbsp. raw cacao powder

- Avocado

- Figs or dates for extra sweetness and fiber

- 1-2 tbsp. nut butter for extra energy and satiety

- Substitute organic milk, goat milk, almond milk, or coconut milk for some of the juice

- Spinach or kale, organic, for an earthy taste

- 2 ounces tofu

- 1 tbsp. wheat germ

Mix together in a high-power blender. This recipe makes 64 ounces. The smoothie tastes best when it's fresh and still has that bubbly milkshake consistency. Refrigerate any leftover smoothie and re-blend before serving later. Sip *slowly* throughout the day.

HOW A SMOOTHIE A DAY KEEPS INFLAMMATION AWAY

Can't wait to get your blender going? Here are seven reasons why this inflammation-balancing smoothie is smart.

Reprograms the gut. The sipping solution part of The Inflammation Solution gets your gut used to a new way of eating by allowing it to be less full, but just as satisfied, with less food at one time. Remember, 70 percent of your immune system lives in the gut, and much of your nervous system resides there, too – the "gut brain." Called *metabolic* *programming,* the sipping solution resets the intestinal tissue back into inflammation balance.

Stabilizes blood insulin. Those three magic words – *stable insulin levels* – have an inflammation-balancing effect. As I noticed my feelings and my energy level becoming more stable, I decided to biochemically check this response by measuring my blood sugar levels every two hours for 48 hours, except while sleeping. They were consistently stable – not too high, not too low. I was avoiding those dreaded spikes as I was reprogramming my gut – and my whole body biochemistry – to get used to this new way of eating and feeling. (See related section, The Hormonal Harmony of Health, page 14.)

Satisfies without being hungry. Don't go hungry! Hunger throws your body more out of balance by prompting you to overeat at the next meal. This is why I experimented with just enough fat, fiber, and protein – high satiety or filling foods – to give me a comfortable gut feeling; not too full, but not hungry, just comfortably satisfied. After a few months of the sipping solution, my gut got used to feeling good. Case in point, when I went to an all-you-can-eat buffet and let my grazing guard down and became a gorger, for the next 24 hours my gut let me know, "You shouldn't have done that!" I felt fatigued and bloated. Gorging now bothers me where previously it didn't. In fact, when a patient with inflammation tells me that a certain inflammation-producing way of eating "doesn't bother me" I say, "It's supposed to bother you. We need to re-program your gut to feel well when you eat

---

POWERFUL POMEGRANATES

Pomegranates are in season during flu season. Thank Dr. Mother Nature – again. Dr. Bill's tip: Quarter a pomegranate so you can scoop out seeds and flesh, and blend them into your smoothie.

well and feel bad when you eat bad." If your gut voice stops prompting you, you're in inflammatory trouble.

Balances inflammation. The inflammation-balancing smoothie, let's call it *inflammation-ade*, is loaded with inflammation-balancing colorful foods, rich in antioxidants, that leverage the powerful healing effect of food *synergy* (see synergy, page 67). If your immune system could talk, it's likely to say, "Finally you are feeding me the foods I need to be in balance."

WHY THE MEDITERRANEAN DIET IS ANTI-INFLAMMATORY

Recent research validates what Mediterranean moms have long preached: the Mediterranean diet of seafood, legumes, fruits, vegetables, unrefined grains, and virgin olive oil has anti-inflammatory effects. What's even more remarkable is that the Mediterranean diet is relatively high in fat (30-40 percent of calories), a food fact that flies against the Western pundits who tout the benefits of low-fat eating. The marvel of the Mediterranean diet is no mystery. It is high in antioxidants. It's simply a real-food, right-fat, and right-carb diet rather than the typical Western way of eating: "low-fat" (translation: high in junk carbs), "fast food" (translation: fast to enter the bloodstream, causing sugar spikes), "fake foods" (translation: chemically modified to help packaged foods last longer but which cause the body to deteriorate faster). The "Medies" eat a lot of vegetables, and will tell you that sautéing them in olive oil and spices makes them taste better so you eat more.

Is the Mediterranean diet nuts? Yes, those you eat. Those who eat low-fat diets often get fatter because they replace real-food fats with fake-food carbs, which don't satisfy enough, so they eat more. Eating more fat (again, a right-fat diet), yet lowering the sticky fats in your blood, flies in the face of the "sweet and low" establishment. This is especially true for the notoriously misguided preaching of low-fat diets for diabetics. Also, dieters are likely to more faithfully stick to the Mediterranean diet because it tastes better than the bland and boring "low-fat" diets.

Reshapes tastes. See the list of all the foods you need to eat – and learn to like – that promote inflammation balance on page 99. Gradually adding these foods (like kale) to your smoothie shapes your tastes toward gradually liking them. Your gut will react to a healthier change in diet by naturally upgrading from, "I don't like it, but must eat it," to "I like it," and eventually to "I crave it." Once you start craving your individual inflammation-balancing diet, you know your body is on the right road to biochemical balance.

Eases heartburn. Because blended food exits from the stomach faster, less food remains in the stomach to get refluxed back up. Heartburn may be the body's natural prompt to sip, dip, and eat less the older we get. In my medical practice, my first "prescription" for healing heartburn is: "Enjoy the sipping solution and graze according to the rule of twos" (see page 117).

SIPPING SOLUTION SUMMARY: WHY IT WORKS

✓ Tastes good

✓ Loaded with antioxidants and anti-inflammatories

✓ Lessens heartburn

✓ Has balanced nutrition: 50-55 percent healthy carbs, 20-25 percent healthy proteins, 20-25 percent healthy fats

✓ Stabilizes blood sugar

✓ Resets the gut to be satisfied with less

✓ Enjoys synergistic effect of many nutrients

You can feel that!

Berry good for your brain. Some of the highest antioxidant levels are found in berries: organic blueberries, blackberries, strawberries, and raspberries.

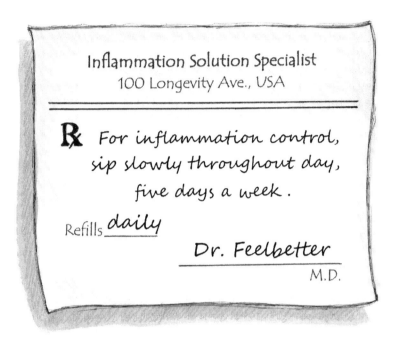

Inflammation Solution Specialist
100 Longevity Ave., USA

℞ For inflammation control, sip slowly throughout day, five days a week.

Refills _daily_

Dr. Feelbetter
M.D.

SALADS

Here are four ways salads are a super anti-inflammatory:

Salads don't spike. Salads (especially greens, nuts, and extra virgin olive oil) blunt the after-meal sticky-stuff spikes (see postprandial lipemia, page 43) that make blood vessels stiff and sticky. The fiber in greens and vegetables slows absorption of sugar and fat – just what your blood vessels need. Because crunchy vegetables, seeds, and nuts require you to eat slower and chew longer, their natural sugars enter the bloodstream more slowly.

Salads are satisfying. Salads enjoy another anti-inflammatory effect called a *high satiety factor*. Salads fill you up so that you become more satisfied with fewer calories. The combination of fiber, healthy fats, protein, and less sticky carbs (also known as low-glycemic index carbs) prompt your body to feel more comfortably full sooner, prompting you to eat a smaller main course (which is usually the part of the meal that's highest in sticky stuff). In fact, we call veggies, nuts, salmon, and extra virgin olive oil "the big-four" foods that are the most satisfying and that contribute the most to inflammation balance, meaning they cause less spikes of sticky stuff in the blood.

Salads enjoy synergy. "Food synergy" is a healing term we want you to enjoy. The more colorful vegetables you put into your salad, the better they work as a team for balancing your inflammation. Note: salads shouldn't swim in dressing.

SAVOR YOUR SYNERGY

One of the healthiest nutritional principles in the six-S anti-inflammatory diet is another "S" – *synergy,* meaning that when you put many of these foods together, such as in a salad or a smoothie, it's like all the forces in your inflammation army get upgraded to behave better, like a biochemical team approach. When you eat many of these antioxidants together, they work in harmony throughout your body and keep your inflammation system in balance. Dr. Mother Nature prescribes synergy in most of her best, food-based anti-inflammatories. Vegetables and fruits have hundreds of antioxidants. Wild salmon also enjoys the synergistic effect of two powerful antioxidants: omega-3s and astaxanthin. So, for the healthiest anti-inflammatory effect, enjoy a *rainbow* of colors in your diet, or as mom said: "Put more color on your plate."

Salads are super-antioxidants. Need some "vegucation?" Let's take a colorful trip through Mother Nature's "farmacy" to see the anti-inflammatory "medicines" that salad ingredients contain.

Greens and beans are a healthful anti-inflammatory team. These are top plant sources of the sticky-stuff lowering nutrient folate, or folic acid, especially asparagus, lentils, spinach, kidney beans, and romaine lettuce.

> **Dr. Bill advises:** Unless your doctor advises otherwise, eat *whole eggs*. For most people, an egg-white omelet makes no nutritional or medical sense.

Add an egg to your salad. Eggs rank close to salmon as one of the most nutrient-dense foods, packing the most inflammation-balancing nutrients per calorie. For a mere 70-80 calories, the egg white is a rich source of protein and the egg yolk contains vitamins A, D, and E. Like salmon, egg yolk is one of the rare foods where vitamin D is naturally found. The yolk is a good source of choline, a vital nutrient for the structure of the cell membranes and cell signaling between brain pathways. Also, lutein and zeaxanthin, the eye-health nutrients, are excellent antioxidants found in egg yolk. And, as an extra nutritional perk, if the hen ate real food (grass, insects, etc.) and not cheap, factory-made food, they may even have a bit of natural omega-3s, DHA and EPA. One of my favorite "snooze foods" is to enjoy an egg before bedtime.

Color	"Medicines"	Anti-inflammatory Actions
Reds: Tomato / tomato sauce Red leaf lettuce Ketchup, organic Watermelon Guava / red plums Red peppers Pink grapefruit Salmon	Beta carotene Lycopene Vitamin C Astaxanthin	Antioxidant Anti-cancer Immune support Inflammation balancing
Yellows: Apricots / peaches Sweet potatoes / yams Pumpkin Carrots Papaya / mango Yellow peppers Squash	Beta carotene Vitamin C Lutein Zeaxanthin	Similar to reds Eye health
Blues / Purples Blueberries Blackberries Grapes Plums Dark cherries, tart	Anthocyanins	Anti-cancer Anti-inflammatory Brain health Heart health
Dark greens Kale Spinach Arugula Romaine Broccoli Asparagus Watercress Chard Collards	Beta carotene Folic acid	Antioxidants Anti-cancer Lowers homocysteine, a very sticky biochemical in the bloodstream.

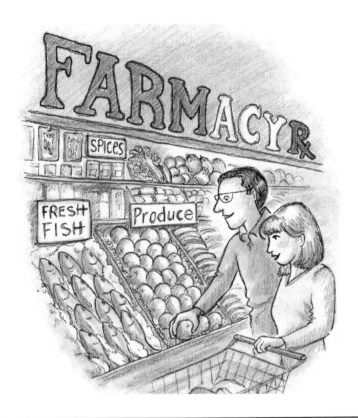

ENJOY DR. BILL'S ANTI-INFLAMMATORY SALAD

- 4 oz. grilled wild salmon fillet
- 3 c. organic greens: spinach, kale, chard
- 1 serving nori (seaweed), chopped
- ½ c. chopped tomatoes
- ¼ cup beans, black or kidney
- 1 tbsp. pomegranate seeds
- 1 tbsp. raw sunflower seeds, walnuts, or pecans
- 1 tbsp. extra virgin olive oil and/or 1 tbsp. hummus
- 1 tbsp. chopped green onions

ENJOY DR. BILL'S ANTI-INFLAMMATORY SALAD (*CONT'D*)

- Juice from half a lemon or lime
- 1 tbsp. goat cheese

Arrange salad ingredients tastefully on a plate. According to your tastes and tolerance, spice it up with grated ginger, turmeric, black pepper, and crushed fresh garlic. Sprinkle with lemon or lime juice and enjoy.

Steam it up! To add variety to your salads *lightly* steam this salad. "Hot salads" are one of my culinary favorites.

SPICES

Spice up your health with Dr. Mother Nature's medicines. Besides adding flavor to your foods, spices are natural anti-inflammatories. I first became aware of the spice effect by observing that patients in my medical practice who ate more spices suffered less "-itis" illnesses. While most spices have anti-inflammatory benefits, here are the, shall we say, most spicy ones.

START LOW, GO SLOW

If you're not already a spice lover, don't overwhelm your taste buds and intestines with a sudden big dose. Start with a few sprinkles and gradually up the amount as your taste buds tell you. I noticed that after a few months, my taste buds and my gut voice welcomed much larger amounts of spices.

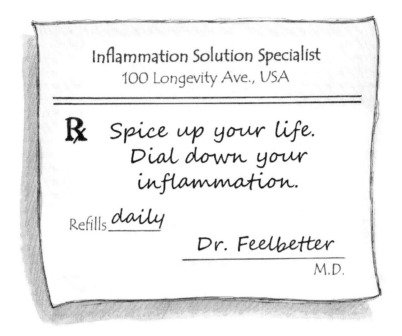

Inflammation Solution Specialist
100 Longevity Ave., USA

℞ Spice up your life. Dial down your inflammation.

Refills *daily*

Dr. Feelbetter
M.D.

Turmeric

Turmeric (curcumin) is the yellow powder from the root of the plant *Curcuma longa*. Turmeric, the yellow spice in curry, has an ancient history as one of Dr. Mother Nature's most respected and researched medicines. Popular in India and Asia where it is a daily staple, in Western medicine, turmeric is gaining what I like to call the AAAA effect: *anti-inflammatory, anti-cancer, anti-coagulant,* and *anti-Alzheimer's.* Here's why science says turmeric is terrific.

Anti-inflammatory effects. Turmeric tames inflammation. It's a natural COX-2 inhibitor, without the uncomfortable side effects those pharmaceuticals have. (See COX explanation, page 12). Although most of the studies have been done in experimental animals, an increasing number of human studies are showing that turmeric behaves as an antioxidant by decreasing the level of sticky biochemicals in the blood, such as oxidized cholesterol, and by generally lowering the level of sticky biochemicals that stick to the lining of the arteries. Remember those painful sounding pro-inflammatory chemicals leukotrienes, thromboxane, prostaglandins, cyclooxygenase 2, tumor necrosis factor, interferon, and interleukin? Research reveals that the levels of all these "hurters" are balanced by turmeric.

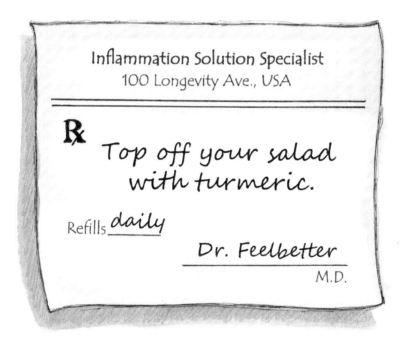

Anti-cancer effects. Turmeric spices up the ability of the immune system to target and kill cancer cells, especially those causing colon cancer. In a fascinating study at the Cancer Research Center of Hawaii, researchers found that the carcinogens in meat cooked at high temperatures (heterocyclicamines) were lower in meat marinated in turmeric-garlic sauce than in meat cooked with barbecue sauce.

Anti-coagulant effects. Turmeric, like fish oil, keeps platelets from becoming too sticky. Researchers discovered that one of the reasons Westerners suffer more cardiovascular disease, especially coronary thrombosis and thrombotic strokes, is that their blood clots too fast (meaning their blood is too sticky). In recent years, cardiologists have discovered that excess fibrinogen, a sticky biochemical naturally found in our blood, may contribute to cardiovascular disease if it gets too high. Of even more concern is the finding that the levels of fibrinogen in the blood increase with age. Turmeric reduces fibrinogen levels.

Anti-Alzheimer's effect. Scientists proved that turmeric crosses the blood-brain barrier and reduces amyloid deposits (sticky stuff) in the brains of experimental animals. This could be one of the reasons that curry-loving cultures, such as India, suffer less neurodegenerative diseases, such as Alzheimer's.

Black Pepper

Most people enjoy the flavor of their daily sprinkle of black pepper without realizing the health benefits of what has been valued since ancient times as "the king's spice." It is one of the oldest treasured "medicines" used by Asian and Indian healers. Like its teammate in synergy, turmeric, black pepper is one of the most studied spices. Here's what science says about how black pepper can enhance your health and heal your hurts.

Enhances digestion. As soon as black pepper hits the taste buds, they send a signal to your intestines to pour out digestive juices, like a "get ready for work" signal. Black pepper is credited with speeding up intestinal transit time. Partially-digested food that lingers too long in your intestines causes a real "pain in the gut," such as heartburn or constipation, and even increases the risk of colon cancer by retaining food residues that cause wear and tear on the intestinal lining.

Eases arthritis and inflammation. As a powerful anti-inflammatory, black pepper has been shown to ease the pain of arthritis. Eating black pepper lessens oxidative stress, especially after eating a high-fat diet.

Enhances absorption. Besides increasing the absorption of turmeric, black pepper increases the absorption of vitamin C. Sprinkle black pepper on your salads.

The nutrient in black pepper that teases your taste buds, triggers the sneezes, and heals your hurts is called *piperine*. Besides enhancing digestion and balancing inflammation, piperine is being studied as a spectacular nutrient to heal other organs, especially those that are vulnerable to inflammation and oxidation, such as the brain.

Tame black pepper with turmeric. One day, I was extoling the virtues of turmeric to one of my patients from India. This smart mom became the doctor, teaching me that Indian medicine has long known

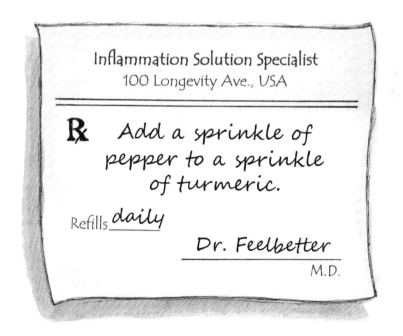

Inflammation Solution Specialist
100 Longevity Ave., USA

℞ Add a sprinkle of pepper to a sprinkle of turmeric.

Refills daily

Dr. Feelbetter
M.D.

that partnering black pepper with turmeric greatly enhances the intestinal absorption of the turmeric, the spice that needs a bit of help getting through the intestinal lining and into the bloodstream. Nearly every time I enjoy a salad, I sprinkle turmeric and black pepper on it. One time just before giving a talk on inflammation, my briefcase fell off a nearby table and out came a tiny package of turmeric. Turning a problem into an opportunity, I mentioned to the audience that after the talk I was going to take my "medicine" (turmeric) into the restaurant, pair it with freshly-ground black pepper, and sprinkle it on a salad topped with salmon.

BETTER PEPPER

Want to make your pepper better? Grind peppercorns in your own peppermill or request freshly-ground pepper in a restaurant. Pepper that is freshly ground retains more of its flavor and health benefits. While still a healthy spice, the longer ground pepper sits around in a shaker, the more flavor it loses and the less piperine it contains. Chefs suggest grinding fresh black pepper into the sauces toward the *end* of the cooking to help it retain most of its flavor. To enhance your health benefits, replace your pepper shaker with a peppermill.

Cinnamon

While I enjoy turmeric and black pepper on my salad each evening, I often sprinkle cinnamon into my oatmeal, smoothie, and café latte. Cinnamon ranks just below honey as my favorite healthy sweetener for these reasons:

Balances blood sugar. Remember, inflammation balance is your health goal. Inflammation balance begins with blood sugar balance.

It's ironic that this sweet spice helps balance blood sugar. Cinnamon is another sticky-stuff-lowering spice. It lowers the level of sticky blood sugars and sticky blood fats like LDL cholesterol and triglycerides, which is why researchers are discovering that cinnamon helps to both prevent and heal type II diabetes. It is noteworthy that this sweet spice has received mixed reviews in the medical literature. Not every study affirms its sugar-balancing effect. Remember HbA1c, the "frosted hemoglobin"? (See page 21) A study published in the *Journal of the American Board of Family Medicine* showed that HbA1c was significantly lower when persons with type II diabetes ate a gram of cinnamon a day. Another study in which type II diabetics ate cinnamon daily did not show a significant change in HbA1c. Can half a teaspoon of cinnamon a day help keep type II diabetes at bay? Probably yes!

Stops sugar spikes, and perhaps also spikes in blood fats or postprandial lipemia (PPL). Remember that bad word in "-itis" illnesses, "spikes"? There is some research showing that cinnamon added to sweet desserts helps reduce their usual sugar spikes. Why the sweet spice may make your blood, shall we say, less sticky, is a subject of interest among spice researchers. The prevailing theory is that cinnamon mimics insulin and makes the receptors in the cells more receptive, or sensitive, to insulin. Scientists at the Human Nutrition Research Center in Beltsville, Maryland, discovered that type II diabetics were able to lower their blood levels of sticky sugars and sticky fats (LDL cholesterol and triglycerides) after eating cinnamon. Cinnamon rolls don't count!

Dr. Bill's sweet tip. Instead of added sugar, try cinnamon in your desserts, coffee, and tea. While certainly less, shall we say, "sweet," I find that cinnamon has a unique sweet flavor that is a sweeter – and healthier – substitute for added sugar. As a colon cancer survivor, I had a personal interest in studying cinnamon after reading a study from one of the top cancer centers – MD Anderson, in Houston, TX

– saying that preliminary research in experimental animals showed that cinnamon inhibited pro-inflammatory pathways in cancer cells, and cinnamon extract inhibited the growth and spread of cancer cells.

HOW TO BUY AND USE CINNAMON

Make cinnamon a sweet "sprinkle" in smoothies, ice cream, and pies. Put pieces of cinnamon sticks in soups, stews, coffee, and tea. In fact, boiling cinnamon sticks in water makes a flavorful and healing tea. Like all the medicines that Dr. Mother Nature makes, the less you mess with them, the more medicinal they are. Like the good word in grains, "whole," the same applies to using spices.

The only downside of cinnamon is the *theoretical* possibility that high doses (3 teaspoons) may drop blood sugar too low in type I diabetics; and because cinnamon contains coumarin, a natural anticoagulant, large doses could theoretically increase the blood-thinning effect of people taking prescription Coumadin.

Dr. Bill's spicy story. I was a bland eater and not really a spice-lover – until I got colon cancer. It was time to practice what I preached – or rather eat what I taught. Part of my personal cancer-prevention program was to survey the best medical studies, and I found the "medicine" spices kept coming up. So I tried to eat as many spices as I could, none of which I was originally fond of. I would sprinkle cinnamon and diced ginger into my smoothie in the morning, and a teaspoon of turmeric and a half teaspoon of freshly-ground black pepper on my salad in the evening. I would periodically sneak in rosemary, chilis, garlic, cardamom, oregano, anise, as well as wasabi mayonnaise on wild rice and crushed garlic in steamed greens. Over a few years, I noticed an intestinal prompt. I gradually went from "don't like, but must eat," to "like a little," to "like a lot," and eventually I began to "crave" these spices. I found I was asking for them when we went out to eat and carrying little packets of spices in my suitcase during travel. The term "spice up your life" took on real meaning for me as I became a believer in the old doctor's tale of the wisdom of the body that teaches: inside your body is a voice that will prompt you to eat what is good for the body and not eat what is bad for it. The more you listen to it, the louder it shouts; the more you don't listen, the quieter it becomes. After years of shutting down my internal voice, I am happier – and healthier – because of finally listening to it.

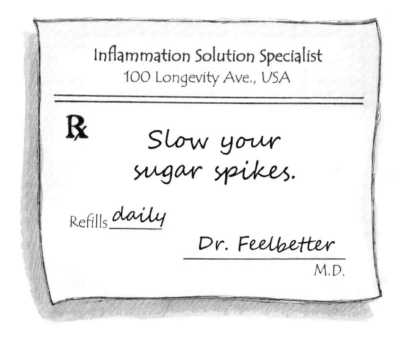

Inflammation Solution Specialist
100 Longevity Ave., USA

R

Slow your sugar spikes.

Refills _daily_

Dr. Feelbetter

M.D.

Chilis

The hotter you eat, the fewer fires, or less inflammation, your body produces. That's why the hotter the chili pepper, possibly the more healing. The anti-inflammatory and pain-relieving nutrient in chili is *capsaicin*. Besides being a natural pain-reliever, chilis contain a lot of antioxidants that quench the fires – and the pain – of excess inflammation.

Chilis are awesome for arthritis. Capsaicin is the top ingredient in topical pain-easing creams. Capsaicin cream applied to knees sore from arthritis has been shown to not only relieve some of the pain, but it may also stimulate the knee joint to produce its own natural anti-inflammatory and lubricating medicines called synovial fluid. Applied topically (but not directly on the sores), capsaicin can soothe the shooting pains from skin viruses like herpes zoster or shingles.

Chilis have anti-inflammatory and possibly anti-cancer effects. I used to shun hot spices because I just didn't like the afterburn in my mouth. After learning about the possible anti-cancer effects of chilis, I started adding chili peppers, such as jalapenos, to my salads in gradually increasing amounts. The wisdom of the body then clicked in. Again, I gradually went from not liking, to liking, to craving hotter spices. And, to my intestinal surprise, there were even studies showing that chilis were good for the gut. My culinary cravings got hotter and hotter – from Cajun food to jerk sauces. I love chopping a spicy jalapeno pepper into tuna fish salad.

If you're a novice at cooking with and eating chilis, be careful! The capsaicin in some potent chilis is volatile and can burn the skin. If your skin is sensitive to chilis, wear plastic gloves and, of course, don't rub your eyes. If you do get a case of "hot mouth" from eating a chili that is too hot, cool the heat with full-fat milk, yogurt, or ice cream. Water won't work and may even make it feel hotter. Same for a skin burn, which can be eased by massaging in a bit of full-fat yogurt, milk, or ice cream.

Ginger

Most mornings I grate into my smoothie a chunk of ginger root about the size of a checker. Our family has treasured the medicinal effects of ginger for many years. My wife, Martha, loved its nausea-easing effects during her seven pregnancies, and it is a family staple to ease seasickness on sailboats. Ginger is great at easing indigestion and heartburn. Later, in my medical practice, I learned that ginger's anti-inflammatory effect is attributed to its nutrient *gingerol*. Try grating ginger into drinks, tea, soups, sauces, and marinades.

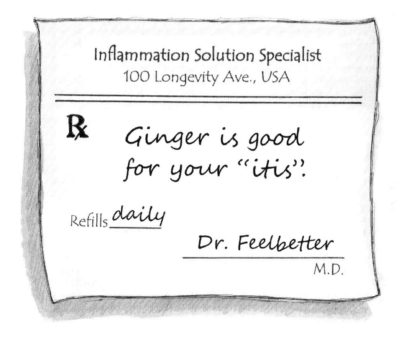

Garlic

To strict foodies, garlic is an "herb," not a spice. The same nutrient in garlic that gives you stinky breath and smelly skin – *allicin* – also is a healing anti-inflammatory. As a medicinal herb, garlic benefits the body from head-to-toe. In this section, we'll just praise the inflammation-balancing effects of garlic:

Makes blood less sticky. Yes, garlic may make your breath stinkier, but it makes your blood less sticky. Remember the story of how sticky stuff causes blood clots (see page 18)? Like many of the spices, garlic makes platelets less sticky. There is also some research evidence that garlic makes blood cells and blood fats less sticky. Studies on the cardiovascular benefits of garlic are mixed – some show benefits, others don't.

Promotes endothelial health. As you learned on page 51, there is special interest in the cardiovascular organ that is the least understood and appreciated, yet one of the most health-promoting systems in your entire body – the endothelium. (Look for my upcoming book on endothelial health called *The Silver Lining*.) Eating garlic nourishes the endothelium, enabling the arteries to not get so stiff. Any nutrient that makes any part of the body less stiff and sticky deserves a place in your anti-inflammatory medicine cabinet.

May reduce the risk of colon cancer. Like the other health-benefits of garlic, its role as a colon-cancer protector seems promising. Even though the science about the health benefits of garlic is somewhat mixed, it definitely belongs in your home medicine cabinet. One of the quirks of garlic that sparked my interest is, while other spices may have variable levels of intestinal absorption, your nose tells you that garlic definitely gets into the tissues of your body. There is certainly no problem with garlic being absorbed. I love it added to guacamole, pesto sauce, mayonnaise, basil, hummus, and diced into steamed salads.

Getting the most "medicine" out of your garlic. Like other spices, the stronger the aroma, usually the more the medicinal effects. Try this test: sniff fresh garlic. Then peel off the paper skin, crush the clove, and sniff how it exudes the aroma. Freshly-crushed garlic has the most medicinal effects. Buy plump bulbs with firm cloves covered with skin, not shriveled. Crushing garlic releases an internal enzyme, allicinase, which forms allicin, the active medicinal ingredient in garlic. Cooking at high temperatures can destroy this enzyme and lessen the medicinal effects.

Other spices having anti-inflammatory effects. While the above spices are the most popular, others deserve honorable mention for their healing, anti-inflammatory effects:

- Anise
- Basil
- Celery seed
- Cardamom
- Cocoa
- Fennel

- Oregano
- Rosemary
- Sage
- Thyme
- Wasabi

(For more information about spices, see Resources, page 267)

SUPPLEMENTS

Continuing with our theme, "show me the science," I have selected those nutritional supplements most supported by scientific studies, those I personally recommend for my patients, and those whose effect on inflammation health I have personally observed. Dr. Bill advises: Enjoy your own personal anti-inflammatory effect by eating these supplements *in addition to*, not instead of, sufficient seafood, fruits, vegetables, and spices.

Omega-3 Fish Oil

We have thoroughly surveyed the science and arrived at this summary of the usual doses for the usual *adult* "-itises". Since you may have a specific inflammation illness, first check with your healthcare provider on the right dose for you*.

HOW MUCH OMEGA-3 FISH OIL SUPPLEMENTS FOR THE HURTS YOU HAVE

Arthritis: 3-4 grams (3,000 mg – 4,000 mg) per day**

Neurological illnesses: 3-6 grams per day

Cardiovascular disease: 1-2 grams per day

Most other illnesses: 2 grams per day, at least

Prevention: 1 gram per day, at least

Pregnant and breastfeeding mothers: 1 gram per day

Infants and toddlers: 300 mg per day

Children: 500 mg per day

Teens: Same as adults

---

* The grams and milligrams listed for each ailment are for the two main omega-3 fats *EPA and DHA*. Read the label nutrition facts and do the math. Add the listed milligrams of EPA and DHA per serving together (e.g., 300 mg EPA plus 300 mg DHA) and adjust the serving size to the right dose (number of capsules or teaspoons) for you.

** For arthritis, science suggests the 3 +3 guideline: 3 grams a day for three months, since it often takes three months to feel improvement.

If you eat *12 ounces of wild salmon* per week, you will get 500-600 mg omega-3 EPA/DHA per day, which is usually sufficient for most healthy adults. If, however, wild salmon is not available to you, or you have a cardiovascular or neurological ailment or "-itis" illness, you will need to take a daily supplement. For more about matching the dose you need with the "-itis" you have, see *The Omega-3 Effect* (Resources, page 267).

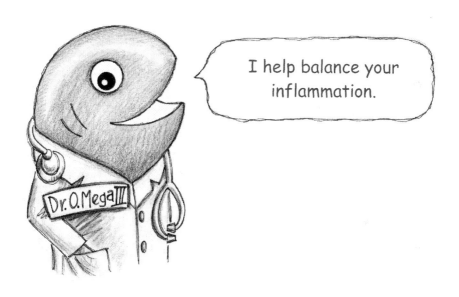

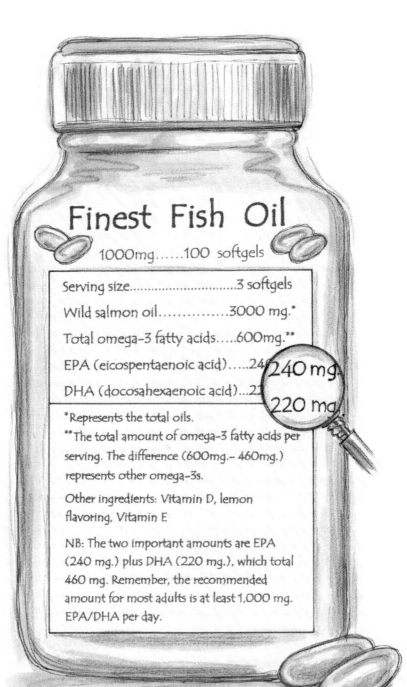

Finest Fish Oil

1000mg......100 softgels

Serving size...........................3 softgels

Wild salmon oil...............3000 mg.*

Total omega-3 fatty acids.....600mg.**

EPA (eicospentaenoic acid).....240 mg.

DHA (docosahexaenoic acid)...220 mg.

*Represents the total oils.

**The total amount of omega-3 fatty acids per serving. The difference (600mg.– 460mg.) represents other omega-3s.

Other ingredients: Vitamin D, lemon flavoring, Vitamin E

NB: The two important amounts are EPA (240 mg.) plus DHA (220 mg.), which total 460 mg. Remember, the recommended amount for most adults is at least 1,000 mg. EPA/DHA per day.

Astaxanthin

The same nutrient that makes seafood so pink is also the one that has a powerful anti-inflammatory effect. Dr. Mother Nature is my most trusted teacher of inflammation knowledge. While fishing in Alaska with my most trusted fisherman, Randy Hartnell, owner of my most trusted seafood source, Vital Choice, I asked Randy, "Why are Alaskan salmon so pink?" Randy replied that the pink pigment, astaxanthin, is nature's most powerful antioxidant. While watching salmon swim upstream, leap over rocks and waterfalls, and literally sprint toward their finish line, I thought if I exercised like that my joints and muscles would get some "-itis," and eventually everything in my body would hurt and nothing would work. Besides, I would wear out long before the race was finished. Enter Dr. Mother Nature. The harder the salmon swim, the redder they get. As they swim upstream to spawn, it's like the salmon open their own internal pharmacy and pop a pink pill – a natural, potent, anti-inflammatory nutrient called astaxanthin. As a nutrient in pink seafood and as a nutritional supplement, astaxanthin is the A-team captain of antioxidants. When you eat wild salmon, you enjoy the synergistic effects of two powerful anti-inflammatories: omega-3s and astaxanthin.

> **Dr. Bill's fish tip: The redder, the better.**

In fact, the more deeply pink, almost red, the salmon, the greater is the anti-inflammatory effect. This colorful fact is why wild Alaskan sockeye salmon is more reddish pink and why it has a higher natural anti-inflammatory effect than the paler farmed Atlantic salmon, which may be colored with synthetic astaxanthin made from petrochemicals.

Among inflammation scientists, astaxanthin is known as one of nature's most powerful tissue-tamers of excess inflammation. As a natural antioxidant in the carotenoid family of nutrients, astaxanthin is known as an inflammation balancer. Its healthful effects are due to its biochemical ability to dial down the overproduction of pro-inflammatories, helping to keep the body in inflammation balance. As a testimony to the age-old "food is medicine" wisdom, astaxanthin works like pharmaceutical anti-inflammatories, but in a more natural and safer way. Like pharmaceuticals, it dials down the COX-2 pro-inflammatory enzymes to keep them from overreacting and damaging the tissue, yet its dialing down is gentler than and not as extreme as the pharmaceuticals. And unlike the anti-inflammatories pharmaceutical companies make, which target only the COX-2 enzyme, astaxanthin, made by Dr. Mother Nature, targets six different inflammatory pathways in a gentler way.

Astaxanthin is also one of the most scientifically-researched, natural, seafood-based anti-inflammatories. Among inflammation researchers, astaxanthin is respected as a healthful "inflamed tissue protector." For example, astaxanthin has been shown to lower the blood level of *inflammatory markers*, biochemicals that are elevated in the bloodstream and give a clue that the inflammatory system is out of balance and dumping too many pro-inflammatories into the bloodstream. Here's a summary of what science says about the awesome *astaxanthin anti-inflammatory effect*:

- Supports the immune system.
- Supports healthy vision.
- Helps protect against dementia.
- Helps protect skin from sun damage.

- Helps balance excessive inflammation.
- Smoothes the endothelium – less sticky stuff.
- Lessens after-exercise "-itis".
- Because it gets into *all layers* of the skin, it has better dermatitis-easing effects than only topical anti-inflammatories.
- Helps balance an excessive inflammation response.
- Experiments show that it crosses the blood-brain barrier and can have neuroprotective effects.

(To learn more about astaxanthin, including how much to eat and where to get it, see Resources, page 267.)

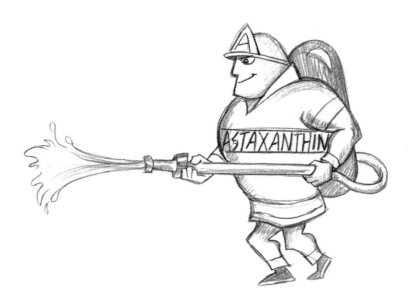

THE COLOR RED

The more color on your plate, the less inflammation in your blood. Which color wins the "Antioxidant Award?" While my personal preference has been the *blue* in blueberries, recent studies suggest the color red may be winning the colorful antioxidant race. For years it was lycopene, the antioxidant that makes tomatoes red and protects them from sunburn; and gives color to pink grapefruit, guava, and watermelon. In the past decade, however, science has uncovered a new red winner – *astaxanthin*. Now sitting at the top of the class of Dr. Mother Nature's most powerful antioxidants, astaxanthin is the natural nutrient that makes salmon pink and red. While lycopene is a plant food, astaxanthin is found in seafood *and* in plant-food, produced by the oldest form of sea life, the sea plant algae. Think, "Astaxanthin comes from algae."

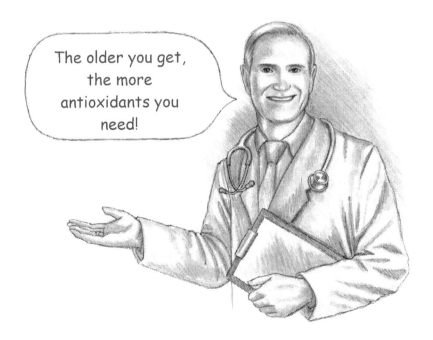

The older you get, the more antioxidants you need!

HOW MUCH ASTAXANTHIN TO HEAL THE HURTS YOU HAVE?

Depending on the severity of your "-itis" illnesses, scientific studies suggest that most people would get the astaxanthin effect they need by eating:

- 4-6 mg of natural astaxanthin a day for prevention and up to 12 mg a day as the upper dosage for severe "-itis" illnesses.

- A generally healthy person without "-itis" illnesses – as prevention: 4-6 mg a day

- Lots of "-itis" illnesses and inflammatory hurts: up to 12 mg a day

These dosages are the ranges in most studies, and natural astaxanthin was found to be safe even at higher doses.

One of the reasons there's such a range of dosages to get the healing effects of food, spices, and supplements is that bioavailability (how much your intestines absorb of what you eat) varies greatly from person to person.

The best seafood source of natural astaxanthin is *wild Alaskan salmon*, which contains around one milligram per ounce, around eight times the amount of astaxanthin found in farmed Atlantic salmon. To get the astaxanthin effect of preventive medicine (4 mg a day), you would have to eat four ounces of sockeye salmon each day, or 1¾ pounds per week. Because most people do not eat that much red salmon, or it's not available to them, natural astaxanthin supplements are recommended. The dose depends on the severity of your "-itis" illnesses. As a show-me-the-science doctor, BioAstin® Hawaiian Astaxanthin is the astaxanthin supplement I recommend in my medical practice because it is the trusted brand that was used in many of the scientific studies. Above all, use natural astaxanthin from sea plants, not synthetic astaxanthin made from petrochemicals. (See

Resources, page 267, for best sources of natural astaxanthin supplements and safe seafood sources).

Spirulina

We doctors trust Dr. Mother Nature's food more than the chemical stuff produced by chemists in the food factory. The closer to nature we eat, the healthier we are. Spirulina not only comes from the most trusted food supplier – the sea – it has the longest history of any food on earth. A nutritional truism we doctors teach is: Eat more *sea*food and more *plant* food. Spirulina, a blue-green algae, enjoys both qualities. It's a *sea plant*. Spirulina is better thought of as a food rather than a supplement. Like the anti-inflammatory effects of omega-3 oils and Hawaiian Astaxanthin, spirulina is *naturally high in inflammation-balancing antioxidants*, especially beta-carotene and zeaxanthin, besides being high in protein and essential minerals and vitamins. As part of your inflammation solution plan, we recommend one teaspoon (3 grams) of Hawaiian Spirulina daily. It's a nutrient for all people at all ages.

I enjoy the head-to-toe health benefits of adding a teaspoonful of Hawaiian Spirulina to my morning smoothie.

Science says spirulina has many healthful qualities, especially:

- Helps build healthy red blood cells and prevents anemia.
- Supports a healthy immune system.
- Supports cardiovascular health by improving blood lipid profiles.
- Has anti-viral activity.
- Helps remove toxic heavy metals and radiation from the body.

(See Resources, page 267 for more about Natural Hawaiian Spirulina.)

POWER UP WITH PHYTOS

Remember the anti-inflammatory wisdom from our mothers: "Put more color on your plate...Eat more fruits and veggies." As always, Mom was right. The inflammation-balancing nutrients in salads and smoothies are called phytonutrients or plant nutrients. "Phytos," for short, give fruits and vegetables their rich color. Phytos are what make tomatoes red, blueberries blue, and spinach green. Plants produce these natural immune-boosting phytos to enable them to survive harsh environments, such as pests and sunburn. You can imagine how "inflamed" a tomato would be from sitting exposed to hot sunshine all day. The red "phyto" lycopene is a natural anti-inflammatory sunscreen. Phyto is a fun term for antioxidants, medicinal biochemicals that plants make to defend themselves, and we eat the plant foods to defend ourselves.

Here's how I explain phytos to kids: "No matter how careful you are to keep germs out of your body, some are going to get in. So, it's important to have a strong army inside you to fight these germs. That germ-fighting army inside you is called your immune system. If your army is strong, it will catch the germs and gobble them up before you get sick; but if it is tired and weak, the germs might win and you get sick. Think of fruits and veggies as 'army food.' The better you feed your army, the better it can fight, and the healthier you'll feel. Also, think of phytos as sports food, such as 'soccer foods,' 'football foods,' 'dance foods,' or whatever you're into. They help your muscles perform better, your eyes see better, and your brain think better. Think of phytos as 'grow foods.'

Go Organic. We can learn so much from Dr. Mother Nature. When we leave a tomato to its natural resources, it builds up its own natural defense mechanisms. My office is only a few feet away from my Tower Garden®, our hydroponic/aeroponic home garden. And most of the tomatoes survive and thrive just fine without outside intervention. Enter the modern tomato in the modern farm. We can't wait patiently for it to grow, thrive, and fill itself with phytonutrients like the organic tomato does. So we spray it with toxins and maybe even protect it from too much sun. Are there any phyto differences between the naturally grown organic tomatoes and the sprayed ones? It's as if the sprayed tomatoes think, "I'm relying on store-bought medicines to protect me so I don't have to make my own." This is why the level of phytonutrients in organically-grown fruits and vegetables is higher than in those that are conventionally grown. Made in my own home *farm*acy, I enjoy one of my favorite anti-inflammatory appetizers: organic home-grown tomatoes on a bed of basil with a drizzle of olive oil and balsamic vinegar and a pinch of turmeric and pepper.

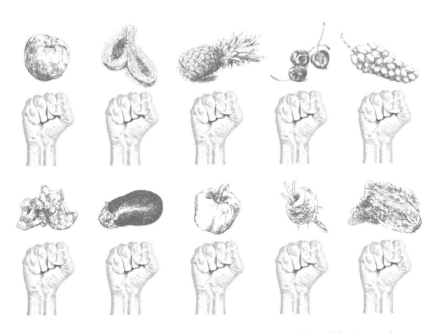

For your inflammation solution, eat 10 fistfuls of fruits and vegetables daily – Doctor's orders!

A phyto night to remember. In 2012, I invited some scientists I called my "phyto friends" to our home for our traditional salmon at sunset dinner. Besides Randy Hartnell, my favorite fisherman, talking about how the phytos in fish are what make salmon pink as you learned on page 87, another guest was Dr. Jeffrey Bland, the father of functional medicine and a leading researcher on the natural effects of phytos on the immune system. From Randy, Dr. Jeffrey, and the other phyto experts, I learned so much about the scientific basis of what mom made me do, "Put more color on your plate." Basically, the way phytos work inside the tomato are to create a sort of biological resilience which programs the genetic machinery of the tomato cell to survive, adapt, and thrive through a variety of harsh environments. Doesn't that sound like the life of many human beings? We want our bodies to be resilient at the cellular level, so when a new germ, environmental stress, or toxin appears, the body can quickly adapt and fight it. Apparently that's what phytos do. They help us adapt and fight. This is why in my office, when talking to children about the importance of eating lots of colorful foods, I draw them a picture of "Phytoman."

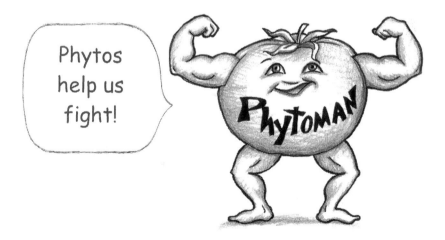

YOUR FARMACY

Dr. Mother Nature prescribes "medicines" that work in a similar, but more selective, way than NSAIDs and which are without side effects. These are phytonutrients. You eat them every day and don't even know it. Next time you're walking through a garden, take a look at a tomato. It sits in the sun most of the day, yet it can't go to the store and slather itself with sunscreen. It's attacked by pests, yet it can't purchase pesticides. So it has to protect itself by mustering up its own inflammatory response to ward off these environmental nuisances so it can bloom into a nutritious and delicious red, ripe tomato. We eat Mother Nature's phytos, or medicines, which helps put our own bodies into inflammation balance. Yes, we could use drugs for this, but not without risk. Mother Nature's pharmacy is without side effects. People don't "overdose" or get rushed to the emergency room because they ate too many salads or drank too many smoothies. Phytonutrients are what gives plants their color, and the physiological reason why mom said, "Put more color on your plate." And for Dr. Mother Nature's medicine, we have the reassurance that these have been tested and perfected over millions of years of tomatoes surviving in their harsh environments; they haven't simply undergone a few years of testing to pass muster with the FDA, which is the case with prescription pills. So you can appreciate this beautiful design: we eat inflammation-balancers, which go into our body and balance our inflammation, and all without prescriptions or side effects.

Phytonutrient researchers have found that the phytos in plant foods work similarly to anti-inflammatory drugs, but they do so in a more selective and gentler way by very *gradually* balancing the immune system, instead of by the quick approach of drugs, which is too strong, and goes on for too long. Most drugs are categorized as *blockers*, meaning they block enzymes within the body and therefore lower the resultant biochemicals that the body produces, such as blocking cholesterol production, acid production, and inflammatory response. The problem is they seldom target only the enzymes they were intended to affect; they also target enzymes we don't want them to touch, thus the "side effect." Phytonutrients, on the other hand, are short-acting and gentle, quickly targeting and regulating enzymes, but not too strong or for too long. In fact, most of the prescription drugs were not tested for long-term use. *You need a personalized plan.*

Cancer caused me to care. As a nearly 20-year cancer survivor who faithfully eats my ten servings of phyto-rich fruits and vegetables nearly every day, I believe that in the near future, we will see targeted therapy for cancer. This means that instead of the shotgun approach to current chemotherapy (when I went through it we called it "nearly killing you and then bringing you back to life"), an individual cancer cell will be extracted from a person with cancer so that a drug can be made to specifically made to attack that cancer cell, but leave the healthy cells alone. Stay tuned!

Fruit and Vegetable Supplements

Most of the illnesses we physicians treat in our medical practices result from a weakened immune system, excess inflammation and poor endothelial function. If you want to prevent, or ease, your "-itises," eat 10 servings (10 fistfuls) of combined fruits and vegetables daily. Since few of us eat that much of Dr. Mother Nature's phytonutrients, the natural medicines that give fruits and vegetables their color, most people wanting to keep their immune system in healthy balance need to take a daily fruit and vegetable supplement. In selecting the best fruit and vegetable supplements, ask yourself the three-S questions:

- Show me the *science*.
- Show me the *synergy*. (Are there over a dozen fruits and vegetables that work as a team?)
- Show me the *safety*.

Specifically, is there science showing that the nutrients in the fruit and vegetable supplement are absorbed into your body? Have there been studies showing that after you take the supplement the blood level of those nutrients goes up? And, is there science showing that once these phytonutrients get into your body, they do healthful things for it? Does it contain only fruits and vegetables? Is it free of chemical additives so it is safe?

The whole food fruit and vegetable supplement I personally take and recommend to my patients is Juice Plus+®. I have always believed that good science and good sense go together. The omega-3, astaxanthin and fruit and vegetable supplements that I recommend basically come from Dr. Mother Nature.

What science says about fruit and vegetable supplements. The health benefits of fruit and vegetable supplements are supported by several published studies in respected scientific journals. A team of researchers from the Department of Nutritional Sciences of the University of Toronto, Canada, published in the October 2011 *Journal of the American College of Nutrition*, analyzed results of 22 studies and found that taking the fruit and vegetable supplement Juice Plus+® boosted immunity, enhanced cardiovascular health, and improved the markers of excess inflammation and endothelial function – primarily by increasing the level of major antioxidants.

Helps inflammation balance. A 2007 study from Tokyo Women's University found that after 28 days on a fruit and vegetable supplement, there was an increase in the blood levels of inflammation balancers (such as beta carotene, lycopene, vitamin E, and folate) and a decrease in the sticky stuff pro-inflammatory markers (homocysteine and lipid peroxides). Researchers at the University of Toronto also found that fruit and vegetable concentrates reduced other inflammatory biomarkers, such as tumor necrosis factor, and showed an increase in some types of normal, protective inflammatory cells, called T-cells.

Like our first two recommended supplements, omega-3 fish oils and natural astaxanthin, fruit and vegetable concentrates reduced oxidative stress in athletes following vigorous exercise. Oxidative stress a form of inflammation, occurs when the body works hard, such

INFLAMMATION-BALANCING FOODS

These foods are our picks for lowering the level of sticky stuff (inflamers) in your blood:

Eat More

Seafood (wild); Astaxanthin; Eggs; Berries: strawberries, blueberries, etc.; Pomegranates; Cherries; Kiwi; Grapefruit (pink); Papaya; Apples; Red grapes; Nuts; Turmeric; Green Tea; Olive oil; Flax oil; Coconut oil; Flax seeds; Ginger; Cinnamon; Chili peppers; Celery; Greens: chard, collards, spinach, kale; Crucifers: bok choy, broccoli, cabbage; Dark chocolate; Garlic; Beans and lentils; Onions; Mushrooms; Sweet potatoes; Nori (seaweed); Wild game: venison, elk; Grains (gluten-free): oatmeal, quinoa; Spirulina (Hawaiian).

Eat Less

Feedlot-fed meats; Chips; Fried foods; Sunflower oil; Safflower oil; Soybean oil; Corn oil; White bread; White pasta; Refined grains.

Eat None*

"Partially hydrogenated" oils; Cottonseed oil **; Canola oil **; High fructose corn syrup; Artificially sweetened beverages; Commercial French fries; Foods containing: monosodium glutamate (MSG, also called "yeast extract" and "hydrolyzed protein"); Artificial colorings, such as red #40

* Highly processed (chemicalized).

** See why, page 141.

as during the vigorous exercise of a marathon runner. Metabolic waste products, called oxidants, can build-up and damage tissues. Eleven clinical studies showed that people who took a fruit and vegetable supplement showed higher blood levels of antioxidants and reduced oxidative stress as evidenced by reduced lipid peroxides, a key indicator of oxidative stress. Studies at both the University of North Carolina and The Medical University of Graz, Austria, showed that in both trained athletes and in healthy exercising volunteers, those who took this fruit and vegetable supplement showed a reduction in markers of oxidative damage to protein and fat resulting from intense exercise, compared to those who didn't.

Vitamin D for Anti-Inflammatory Defense

While it's best to get sufficient amounts of this anti-inflammatory from Dr. Mother Nature – *salmon and sunshine* – many people with "-itis" illnesses have a vitamin D insufficiency. There are two modern reasons for this. The first is that most of us are not twice-weekly salmon eaters (a six-ounce fillet of wild salmon contains around 4000 IU of vitamin D). By the way, salmon has a triple-A effect as an anti-inflammatory food: omega-3s, astaxanthin, and vitamin D. The second is that we are a generation of sun phobics, failing to expose our skin to the sun for the recommended 15-20 minutes a day. I call it the "indoor disease." Be sure your blood vitamin D level is part of your inflammatory profile when your doctor measures it. (See Measuring Your Markers, page 238.) A 2014 study showed that correcting low vitamin D levels can result in a lowering of the inflammatory markers (sticky biochemicals) in the blood.

Vitamin D is vital. Very simply, vitamin D insufficiency – another antioxidant or anti-sticky stuff deficiency – affects the majority of inflamed persons. (To be chemically correct, vitamin D is a *hormone* more than a vitamin.) Cell biologists rate the importance of antioxidants and other nutrients by the number of receptors they have on the cell membranes. Modern technology allows windows into the cell, revealing "doors" or reserved "parking places" on cell membranes called receptors. The more receptors on the cell membrane, presumably the more the cell needs these nutrients, sort of like the cell is saying: "Vitamin D delivery trucks, park here and unload your nutrients." Vitamin D researcher, Dr. Michael Holick, values this vitamin so much that he calls it the "D-delightful solution for health." The optimal blood level of Vitamin D is above 50 ng/mL.

As a general guide, you need to take 100 IU of Vitamin D per day for each 1 ng/mL you need to raise your level to reach 50. For example, if your measured Vitamin D level is 30 ng/mL, you should take or eat an additional 2,000 IU per day with the fattest meal of the day, since some fat is necessary for optimal vitamin D absorption. Six ounces of salmon gives you around 4,000 IU of vitamin D. Fifteen minutes of warm-weather sunshine in a swimsuit gives you roughly 5,000-10,000 IU, depending on several factors including latitude, time of day, skin tone, and so on. Because persons vary greatly in their ability to make and metabolize vitamin D, one person may need more sunshine, salmon, and supplements than another person.

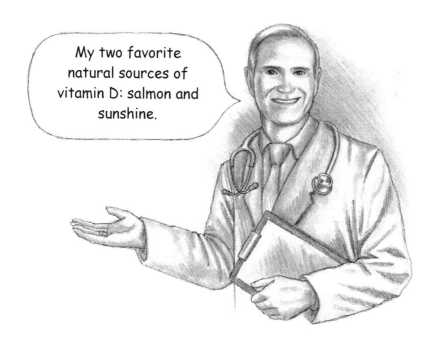

My two favorite natural sources of vitamin D: salmon and sunshine.

Probiotics

Put the best bugs in your bowels. You've heard of probiotics, the bacteria found in yogurt. These good bacteria naturally inhabit the intestines and, in return for a warm place to live, they do healthful things for the body. New research reveals that the immune cells in the gut, or *inflammation regulators*, and the resident intestinal bacteria enjoy a cross-talk of inflammation language. They prompt these gut inflammation police to dial up pro-inflammatories to suppress infection and dial down their fight to prevent excess inflammation or "-itis", such as colitis and inflammatory bowel disease. Probiotics prompt healthy *flora*, the medical term for planting a good garden in your gut. Feed your gut garden good food and you get good bacteria growing there. These beneficial bacteria are picky eaters. The more natural the food you eat, the more naturally your bowel bugs behave. Feed it junk food and your gut garden doesn't grow healthy bacteria. The right intestinal bacteria are the best buddies the gut police have. These probiotic bacteria sort of patrol the lining of the gut and alert the gut police (the immune cells lining the intestines) that foreign germs got in. One of the newest good-gut teachings: to transform the health of your gut, you have to have *the right mix of microbes*. (See more about probiotics for babies, page 247.)

Are you ready for some "wow!" research? Not only do these friendly and healthful bacteria talk with the gut brain police to protect the lining of the gut from inflammation, these lovely little bugs communicate with the head brain to help healthy behavior. One of the most exciting areas of research is the correlation between what's going on in the gut brain and how it affects behavior in the head brain.

WHAT NOT TO EAT: HOW FAKE FOOD INFLAMES YOUR BODY

In a nutshell, the anti-inflammatory diet is a real-food diet. Real foods are those that go directly from a farm or forest, off a tree, out of the ground, or from the sea – and into our mouths. They spend little or no time being processed in a food factory. Here's where good science and good sense match. The inflammation system in your body has adapted over thousands of years to conclude, every time you put food in your mouth: "This is real food for real health. It fits the natural biochemistry of the body. It is welcome here, so we won't fight it. In fact, we'll escort it throughout the body and help the body use the food healthfully." Medically the "real food effect" is called *metabolic programming*. Real foods program the cells to perform the way they were designed so that they balance inflammation.

Then comes along a potato or piece of chicken that once was a real food. To make the food cheaper and last longer on the shelf (but make your *body* more expensive in health costs and not last as long), the food biochemists alter these real foods and make them unreal. Your body's inflammation system is a picky eater. It doesn't recognize some French fries or chicken nuggets as real food, so it gives a different inflammatory response. The inflammation system concludes: "This fake food doesn't fit here. I'll fight these fake foods." This inflammatory fight causes the build-up of sticky stuff – an inflammation imbalance – and you get an allergy or "-itis." We are a country where food costs are lower and medical costs are higher. Any correlation?

Think of food entering the body like a new kid in the neighborhood. If the kid is friendly, he is welcomed into the group and a healthy camaraderie occurs. Suppose a bully (fake fat or carb) enters. Because the bully doesn't fit in, the rest of the kids fight him (inflammation).

Inflammation researchers believe that the more chemical-sounding the ingredient list in the fake food, the more the body's defenses fight it and the more inflammation it causes. Feed your inflammation army many healthy foods and they can fight a healthy fight (wellness). Feed them unhealthy foods and they fight unhealthfully (illness). Fake foods all have one harmful effect in common: they cause fat and/or sugar *spikes* in your bloodstream. Here are everyday examples of how fake foods inflame and infect your body.

THE FRENCH FRY EFFECT

Let's follow those problem potatoes from the frying pan into the fire and see how this fried stuff ignites the fires in your body. The same chemical mischief that makes a fry crispy also makes your body, shall we say, crispy. Here's how frying the oil fries your body: First, the cooking oil starts out unhealthy. To make it last longer for re-use, restaurants often use a mutant oil, called hydrogenated oils, and they re-use it, which mutates it even more, each time increasing its levels of artery-clogging inflammatory fats.

The fries cooked in unhealthy oil are made even unhealthier by the heat attacking them, causing even more chemical mischief. Frying high-carb foods at high temperatures produces a "sticky" chemical called *acrylamide* (sounds like something you don't want in your body). Those fried fries now start frying your body. First stop, your tongue and taste buds, unfortunately the weakest part of your body's defense system. After years of eating French fries, your taste buds have been reprogrammed to accept these foreign foods and even start to crave them: "Ah, the mouth feel of fried fat!" Dr. Mother Nature intended us to get a mouth feel for good fats, not bad fats.

After the sticky fries slide through the mouth, they go into the gut. Your gut is a picky eater. When foreign food enters it, it says, "You don't belong here. We're going to kick you out." Dr. Mother Nature, knowing that most of our inflammatory problems would enter our bodies through the gut, made the gut the largest component of your body's immune system, containing around 70 percent of the immune-response tissue in your body. I call the lining of the gut a *silver lining*. When the gut police of your immune system identifies the fries as a fake food, a fight breaks out, called an *inflammatory response*. When the intestinal lining fights fake food, the battle in the intestinal lining results in debris left over and creates a messy battle ground. The intestinal lining eventually gets injured (colitis, irritable bowel syndrome, and other intestinal inflammatory disorders) resulting in a chronic pain in the gut.

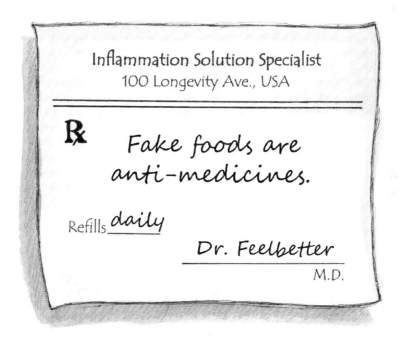

Inflammation Solution Specialist
100 Longevity Ave., USA

℞ Fake foods are anti-medicines.

Refills *daily*

Dr. Feelbetter
M.D.

Medically called the *inflammatory cascade*, one "-itis" leads to another. While the intestinal police do a good job of fighting foreign germs like bacteria – millions of years of genetic training have equipped them to do this effectively – molecular misfits in the chemical foods like the fake fat-soaked French fries fool the gut police, who have had only a hundred years or so to train for this modern cuisine. A hundred years ago, food was farm to fork and, like early airport security, the gut police weren't that threatened. Nowadays, farm food makes detours through a food factory and gets both chemicalized, to last longer, on the shelf and flavor-enhanced. This process, dubbed "food doping," causes us to overeat and overbuy, earning weighty profits for the food factories. While real food was recognized by the body as a non-threat and passed right through the intestinal security screening without much fuss, the fake food is recognized as foreign, a fight breaks out in the gut lining, and an "-itis" illness develops

More "-itis" illnesses downstream. Some of the foreign enemies in the fake food, the ones with long chemical names, such as butylated (sounds like mutilated) hydroxyanisole, get through intestinal security, into the airport, and onto the planes of the body – your bloodstream. Here's where the "global threat", or total body inflammation, begins.

When those mutant chemicals reach your arteries, watch out. The sticky stuff that made it through intestinal security starts to stick to the lining of your arteries, your endothelium, like tar spilling on a smooth highway, causing a dreaded disease you'll hear more about in Chapter Four – *endothelial dysfunction*.

Eat fries – fry your arteries. Not yet convinced to eat your last fast-food French fry? Here's what science says. Fat researchers, I mean scientists who study the effects of fats on our health, fed young volunteers typical restaurant French fries and tested the eaters' arteries before and after this fatty assault. Before the fries, the subject's arteries were soft and flexible. It is the hallmark of healthy arteries to be able to get wider and narrower to accommodate the changing needs for blood flow, such as during rest and exercise, like a highway that would automatically widen during rush hour traffic. After the French fry effect, their subjects' arteries were temporarily stiffer and less likely to accommodate changes in blood flow. Called endothelial dysfunction, stiff arteries are the underlying contributor to cardiovascular disease. Eating French fries regularly makes the arteries stay stiff, and leads to high blood pressure, heart attacks, and stroke. If your inflammation system could talk it would advise, "To keep from getting real sick, just eat real foods."

Avoid "burger brain." One day while playing golf with noted neurologist and Alzheimer's authority Dr. Vincent Fortanasce, we discussed the brain effects of the chemical combo burger and fries. Dr. Vince passionately targeted this combo as leading to "burger brain" because the trans fats cause the blood level of the other sticky stuff chemicals to go even higher. Unlike the principle of good food synergy you learned on page 67, combining these "anti-medicines" increases their unhealthful effects, especially on the brain.

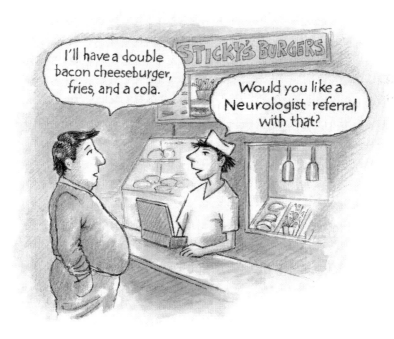

THE CHICKEN NUGGET EFFECT

Still not convinced that fake food causes your hurts? Imagine what your wisely-selective inflammatory system thinks when you eat chicken nuggets, whose ingredients read like a chemistry chart:

Ingredients: White boneless chicken, water, food starch – modified, salt, chicken flavor (autolyzed yeast extract [aka: MSG], salt, wheat starch, natural flavoring [botanical source], safflower oil, dextrose, citric acid, rosemary), sodium phosphates, seasoning (canola oil, mono- and di-glycerides, extractives of rosemary). Battered and breaded with: water, enriched flour (bleached wheat flour, niacin, reduced iron, thiamin mononitrate, riboflavin, folic acid), yellow corn flour, food starch – modified, salt, leavening (baking soda, sodium acid pyrophosphate, sodium aluminum phosphate, monocalcium phosphate, calcium lactate), spices, wheat starch, whey, corn starch. Prepared in vegetable oil (may contain one of the following: canola oil,

CHEMICAL CUISINE

Eating out may be hazardous to your inflammation health. During a recent stay at a chain hotel where breakfast is included in the room price, I hungrily entered the breakfast room. There should have been a sign: "Enjoy a chemical breakfast." I noticed the "lite" yogurt, which means light on nutrition and heavy on added chemicals; chemically-packaged egg omelets, recognized by the fact that they are all identical shapes and sizes; instant oatmeal, which means the nutrients that take time to cook have been removed; and artificially-colored, flavored, chemically sweetened, and taste-enhanced cereals and pastries. I couldn't resist the opportunity to thank the restaurant manager for giving me material for this book. Can you imagine how hotel breakfasts could be upgraded if every guest, when booking their stay, would inquire, "Do you serve a *real* or *chemical* breakfast?"

corn oil, soybean oil, hydrogenated soybean oil with TBHQ and citric acid added to preserve freshness), dimethylpolysiloxane added as an antifoaming agent)

UNSWEETEN YOUR INFLAMMATION

Research is revealing what doctors have long suspected: artificial sweeteners added to beverages, such as high fructose corn syrup, can throw the body out of inflammation balance by increasing the level of sticky stuff in your blood (oxidative stress) and by lowering blood antioxidant levels. Even artificial sweeteners added to diet sodas (sucralose, aspartame) may trigger inflammation. The immune system seems to reject these chemicals as foreign to the body and reacts to them (DrSearsWellnessInstitute.org/resources/inflammation/sweeteners).

THE COLA EFFECT

Your immune system doesn't like sugar surges, especially fake chemical sugar surges. When the body is in biochemical balance, such as stable blood sugar, the inflammatory response system tends to be stable, or balanced. But when the blood level of sugar molecules is too high, such as after guzzling a 24-ouncer, the body believes, "This is foreign to my health" and fights this sugar spike. The resulting mess is called "adhesion molecules" (i.e., sticky stuff that adheres to the lining of your blood vessels, making them stiff). According to an article in the May 2013 issue of *Life Extension*, our national food stamp program pays billions of dollars for soft drinks every day. That's not smart!

THE STEAKHOUSE EFFECT

One of the most tragic sticky stuff stories I have encountered is when my friend John nearly died of a massive heart attack after downing a big steak at a steakhouse. Cardiologists dub this correlation the *steakhouse syndrome.*

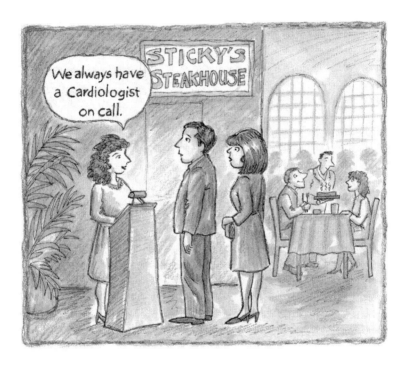

After you eat a high-fat meal, such as a marbled steak with a butter-based sauce, your arteries go berserk, as if to say, "How could you do this to us?" The blood goes into a *hyper-sticky state,* or sludging, and the vessels constrict, or harden – both of which lessen blood flow to the vital organs. The fats in the blood go way up and blood pressure also tends to rise. Also, fibrinogen levels go up. Fibrinogen is an element in the blood that is important for normal blood clotting. The fat particles from the meal traveling around the bloodstream adhere to the fibrinogen, causing millions of tiny thrombotic molecules – sticky stuff – to travel throughout the bloodstream, gradually clumping together and forming blood clots. This can lead to coronary thrombosis (heart attack) or stroke.

Also, high blood fats following a high-fat meal (medically known as *postprandial lipemia* cause the endothelium to release substances that constrict the arteries and cause the blood to get sticky and become prone to clot. A big, high-fat meal causes big fat damage to the blood vessels. Called food energy toxicity (see page 45), the circulating fats continue to irritate the lining of the blood vessels, causing them to get hard and clogged. As you learned on page 54, the smooth omega-3 oils found in seafood blunt this effect, unlike the sticky oils in steak.

The triple threat to inflammation. One day I drove by a fast-food joint and noticed a big ad for a big meal: fries, chicken nuggets, and a cola. "Where have the real foods gone?" I lamented. There should be cardiology clinics set up next to these sticky restaurants.

WHITE IS WRONG FOR INFLAMMATION BALANCE

There is an inflammation health slogan coming to a preventive medicine doctor's office near you: "White out your eating!" Real wheat is not naturally white. Do white bread and white pasta harm your health? These usually factory-processed foods have a high glycemic index, meaning they cause high sticky sugar spikes – glycation – in your blood. "White out" is one of the current, anti-inflammatory buzzwords, and refers especially to white bread. (See related topic, Avoid Spikes, page 43.)

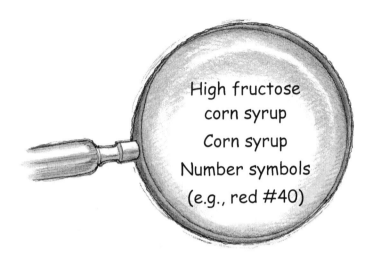

High fructose
corn syrup
Corn syrup
Number symbols
(e.g., red #40)

Look for sticky words on food labels.

WHAT'S WRONG WITH WHEAT? THE EPIDEMIC OF GLUTEN SENSITIVITY

There's a lot of grain blame going on. Wheat "-itis" books, such as *Wheat Belly* and *Grain Brain*, have educated readers about the hidden health-harming inflammatory effects of unreal wheat.

Dr. Bill's supermarket wheat lesson: I take my kids and grandkids shopping and use the supermarket as a giant nutritional classroom. Try this loaf lesson: Have your child pick up a loaf of white bread (I call it "airbread") in one hand and a loaf of 100 percent whole-wheat bread (I call it "grow bread") in the other. Ask your child if she feels any difference. When your child squeezes the white bread you'll probably get an answer like: "It feels squishy" or a kid-only word I love – "smushy." When they squeeze the 100 percent whole-grain bread, they usually say it feels "heavier" or "firmer." I then ask the sports-minded kids: "Do you want your muscles to feel weak and squishy like the white bread, or firm and strong like the whole-wheat bread?" They get it. "Enriched," on a bread label often means "deprived of nutrients." I once did the revealing math. Enriched means the food chemists took out many of the richer nutrients that might spoil faster and "impoverished" the bread with cheaper chemical ingredients. Most white bread could be called "iBread," or inflammation bread.

An example of the unreal food effect is the rising epidemic of *gluten sensitivity*, another gut "-itis." The prevailing theory is we are no longer eating real wheat (nor real corn or real soy). Because the genetic make-up of these foods has been changed, the body no longer recognizes them as real foods and attacks them. An example of the modern wheat "-itis" connection is the possible correlation between gluten sensitivity and autoimmune thyroiditis and even cognitivitis and Alzheimer's disease.

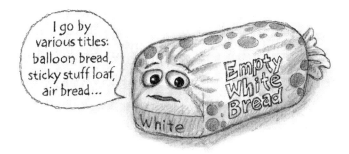

A grain-drain story. A generally health-conscious family in my practice began having unexpected medical problems. Dad and child were growing bigger bellies despite careful eating. Mom developed signs and symptoms of thyroid disease. Many blood tests and specialist consultations later, gluten sensitivity was the suspected cause. Within six weeks off gluten, the male bellies leaned out and mom's thyroiditis lessened. The prevailing explanation of the relationship between gluten sensitivity and thyroid disease is that in some persons the

A TALE OF TWO FUELS

As I was pumping gas into my car, I noticed the gas station's ad touting their clean fuel: "Low quality gasoline can leave *crud* on your engine parts. Take care of your car and it will take care of you." Same for our body. Low quality or fake food leaves crud (sticky stuff) on your body parts. Take care of your body and it will take care of you.

Why we eat. Food benefits our body in two ways: it *fuels* and *heals*. Calories provide fuel for our body's engine. Food provides healing nutrients that grow and repair tissues, explaining the ancient wisdom that food is medicine. Notice how we began getting real sick once we replaced real foods with fake foods.

Real food is clean fuel. It burns "clean." It doesn't gum up the body's engine with crud or "sticky stuff." It has just the right "octane," or calories, to keep you lean and satisfied, but not too much so you get sick and fat. Real food heals because it is high in nutrients that dilute the exhaust produced by burning fuel. Real food balances calorie-burning with tissue wear and tear and repair. The body stays in balance.

Fake food burns "dirty fuel" and hurts instead of heals. "Processing" removed the balance between calories burned and tissues healed. By adding more junk calories, but removing healing nutrients, here's what happened to health.

Fake food causes too much fuel. By adding chemical "flavor enhancers," you eat more fuel than the body needs. The body stores this excess fuel by building a bigger fuel storage tank – a bigger belly – *strike one!*

Fake food burns dirty fuel. It produces exhaust faster than the body can remove it because the exhaust removers have been processed out. *Strike two!*

Fake food lacks healers. Food chemists processed out the healers (phytonutrients, antioxidants) and processed in *anti-healers*, such as MSG, high fructose corn syrup, and so on. *Strike three!* You're out of health.

immune system gets confused, thinks the gluten molecules and the person's own thyroid tissue are the same and attacks both. Stories such as this have changed me from a gluten sensitivity skeptic to a believer.

CHAPTER 3

Twelve Simple Ways to Eat the Anti-Inflammatory Way

Now that you've learned what to eat, it's equally healthful to know how to eat. The anti-inflammatory way of eating means not only keeping sticky stuff out of your mouth as much as possible, but also keeping the level of sticky foods that do get into your gut from getting too high in your blood. In putting together my healthiest list of inflammatory-balancing foods and ways to eat, I first selected criteria for putting together the anti-inflammatory way of eating:

Show me the science. I don't put any food into my mouth, or recommend it to my hurting patients, if it isn't backed up by solid science. The field of nutrition is rife with fads and junk science making faulty conclusions motivated more by money and marketing than by solid science. This is why I've included over 100 scientific references beginning on page 268.

Consider the source. Can you trust government guidelines? Sometimes. The government is still suffering indigestion from approving trans fats and its original food pyramid, known in medical circles as the Titanic Food Pyramid, which will go down in history as the most unhealthy dietary advice ever given. It was prompted by politics and special interest lobbying rather than the best interests of the health of American people. Most nutritionists have a fix for the original U.S. Department of Agriculture (USDA) food pyramid: "Just turn it upside down so refined carbs are sparsely at the top and healthy fats are prominent at the base." Although the revamping of the food pyramid (www.MyPlate.gov) is certainly an improvement, there is a major flaw that, until corrected, will always make government guidelines hard to digest: food guidelines are made by the USDA, which is infected with special interest Big Food and Big Farm groups, instead of by the National Institutes of Health (NIH), the most trusted scientific health department of the U.S. government. I had the privilege of spending two years in research at the NIH and had a dream that if I could be surgeon general for an hour, the first change I would make would be to shift responsibility for all food guidelines from the USDA to the NIH. Still dreaming!

Here are time-tested and science-based eating tips to balance your immune system:

1. GRAZE

Keep your body in inflammation balance. *Graze* on frequent mini meals of healthy food throughout the day instead of gorging on fewer large meals. Why? Simply put, grazers get less sticky stuff in their blood and tissues than do gorgers.

Enjoy Dr. Bill's anti-inflammatory rule of twos. During an average day in my medical office, I "recommend" this memorable anti-inflammatory tool, especially for my patients with the "shuns" – inflamma*tion*, indiges*tion*, and constipa*tion*.

- Eat *twice* as often
- Eat *half* as much
- Chew *twice* as long
- Take *twice* the time to dine

You can do that!

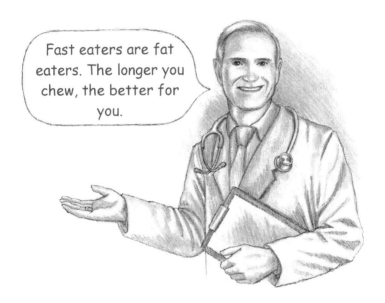

Fast eaters are fat eaters. The longer you chew, the better for you.

Use chopsticks. Forget the fork and use chopsticks. Chopsticks force you to take smaller bites, eat more slowly and better enjoy each bite. You'll feel fuller sooner and are less likely to overeat. We tried this experiment in our family and medical practice and it's one of the most useful weight-management strategies, in addition to helping you enjoy the after-meal good gut feelings. And as an added cerebral perk, the new fine motor movements help you grow new brain pathways.

My Japanese good-gut feeling experience. While writing this book, I had the privilege of lecturing at a scientific meeting in Japan. During my trip, I ate more but felt more comfortable after the meals. Why? I wondered. I concluded that there were three reasons:

1. Using chopsticks prompted me to take smaller bites and take a longer time to dine.

2. The food was real, not processed, such as seafood, tofu, vegetables, and lots of spices like ginger. All these foods give you less of a spike in blood fats and less uncomfortable full feelings after a meal.

3. Sipping green tea with the meal helped blunt the spikes.

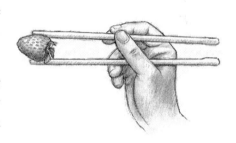

The Japanese have fewer inflammatory diseases, probably because they put less sticky stuff in their mouths in the first place.

THE HORMONAL HARMONY OF GRAZING

Think of your body as a giant biochemical orchestra and each hormone as a player. When all the hormones, especially the inflammation hormones, are in balance, beautiful music, or wellness, results. When the hormones are out of balance – meaning one plays too loud, another plays too soft, or one plays too strong for too long – your body is in inflammation imbalance, or illness. Grazing gives you *stable insulin levels* – the three magic words of hormonal harmony. Think of insulin as the master conductor of your hormonal symphony. When your insulin is stable ("on key"), the rest of the inflammation players in your orchestra are in hormonal harmony and your body plays beautiful music. Your body is in balance!

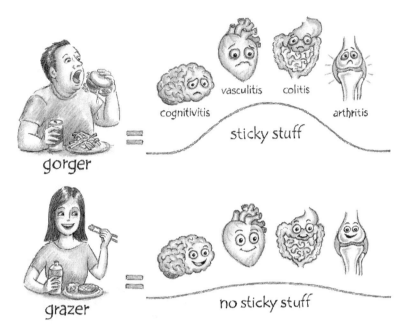

cognitivitis   vasculitis   colitis   arthritis

gorger   =   sticky stuff

grazer   =   no sticky stuff

A Tale of Two Eaters

George the Gorger vs. Gracie the Grazer

To understand why Gracie's body enjoys inflammation balance and George's does not, let's follow both of these eaters from mouth to joints to understand why grazers hurt less and gorgers hurt more. Another way to look at the difference between grazers and gorgers is that gorgers have more "sticky-stuff spikes" in their blood and grazers have fewer. Sticky-stuff spikes are the root cause of many inflammatory flare-ups. To get your body back into inflammation balance, try to remember each time you eat, "no spikes." If your immune system could talk, it would prompt you, "No sticky-stuff spikes, please."

George the Gorger. George's nickname is "Spikey" because he gets a lot of high-fat and sugar spikes in his blood. He eats SAD – the Standard American Diet. George feasts on all-you-can-eat buffets. As he gazes longingly at the array of food, his brain is already in inflammatory trouble. He may not know it, but digestion begins in the brain – called the *cephalic phase of digestion.* Just the anticipation of all that tasty food gets the digestion juices – and the inflammatory biochemicals – turned on. George is in inflammatory trouble even before he takes his first bite. George grabs a giant plate and proceeds to the steak section where he prompts the griller, "Bud, burn a big one for me!" Next to the sticky sirloin he puts a big scoop of buttery mashed potatoes slathered with creamy gravy. Then he scarfs down a big bowl of pasta with Alfredo sauce and fries and chases these sticky fats with a cola. The level of unhealthful saturated fats are so high in his bloodstream that they saturate the endothelium with sticky stuff. During this sticky meal, the blood vessels get so upset they actually start quivering – called vasospasm, or narrowing. The blood level of sticky fats (called postprandial lipemia) and sticky sugars (called postprandial glycemia) goes sky high. Blood flow goes into a hyper sticky state, called sludging, causing the blood vessels to get narrower and blood flow to slow. The sticky stuff, in effect, causes a traffic jam, which can result in a blood clot, coronary thrombosis, or stroke.

Within a couple hours after this high-fat meal, sticky fats, or triglycerides, go up. Another sticky chemical called fibrinogen also goes up. Fibrinogen is like a fishnet of chemicals that help your blood clot. A certain level of fibrinogen is necessary to help your blood clot in case you cut your finger. However, too much causes the blood to clot too fast. (See related subject, The Steakhouse Effect," page 110.)

A little known nutrifact is that when you combine junk carbs with burnt meats this combo causes sticky blood sugar levels to remain higher for longer, doing double damage.

Meanwhile, down in the joints: If George's blood vessels survive the gorging, the inflammatory chemicals have been turned so high that the "-itis" dial gets turned up, resulting in a total body inflammatory effect. Fewer organs work and more organs hurt. The blood cells can't flow as quickly because there's a lot of sticky stuff floating around to slow them down. The SAD diet sets George up for a SAD life (sick all day).

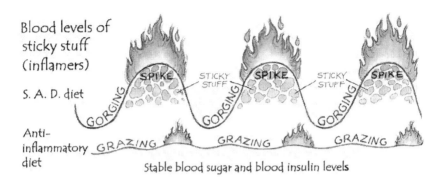

Gracie the Grazer. Gracie's nickname is "Steady" because her blood levels of fats and carbs are steadier than those of "Spikey" George. Gracie frequents a restaurant that specializes in Asian cuisine and also has a delectable salad bar. Her eyes zero in on the salad bar first because her brain tells her – as her mother always did – that beginning a meal with a salad gets her blood level of anti-sticky-stuff biochemicals (antioxidants) high to protect her blood vessels and tissues from too much sticky stuff getting into them too fast. Gracie sits down with a small plate of salad in one hand and chopsticks in the other. She slowly grazes on the salad, chewing each small bite 20-30 times, and enjoying a humorous conversation between bites. She goes back for seconds, again with a small plate, and enjoys a salmon fillet, grilled asparagus, and some wild rice. Gracie's tummy feels full and satisfied because she chews each bite carefully, stimulating more saliva, her body's natural intestinal-health juice to pre-digest the food even before it reaches her stomach. If her blood vessels could talk they

GRAZERS VS. GORGERS	
Grazers are...	**Gorgers are...**
• Likely to be more lean	• More likely to be fat
• More satisfied, less hungry	• More hungry, less satisfied
• Clearer thinkers	• Foggier thinkers
• Less moody	• Likely to have mood swings
• More alert	• Sleepier
• More energetic	• Less energetic
• Have comfortable gut feelings	• Have pains in the gut
• Have fewer "-itis" illnesses	• Have more "-itis" illnesses

would say, "Thank you, Gracie, our traffic is flowing smoothly during the after-meal rush hour." Her choice of salmon vs. sirloin is also good for her gut and blood vessels. The omega-3s in the salmon increase the enzyme lipoprotein lipase (LPL), which helps clear these sticky fats, triglycerides, from her bloodstream. (After a salmon meal, you don't get the postprandial lipemia response that happens after scarfing down a steak. Unlike the steak fats that stick to the blood cells and slow them down, the smooth fats in the salmon ride along on the surface of the blood cells and make them less sticky so the traffic doesn't slow after the meal.)

When Gracie bypasses the meat counter and goes directly to the seafood and salad section, unlike George, she likely avoids a coronary bypass. Studies show that the steak effect and the seafood effect are very different regarding postprandial lipemia, which doesn't occur after a seafood meal as opposed to a dangerously fatty meat meal. Think sticky steak versus smooth seafood. As another postprandial perk, a seafood-rich meal causes more postprandial satiety, also called "after-meal fullness," enabling the eater to feel more comfortably full sooner. Gracie's diet of eating real food real often helps her feel real good.

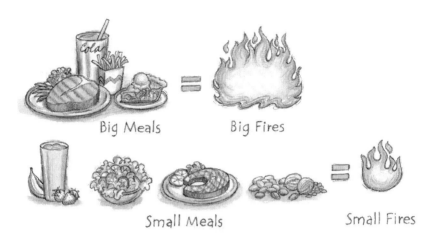

Big Meals   Big Fires

Small Meals   Small Fires

2. SMALLER BITES GIVE SMALLER SPIKES

Not only does eating less sticky food give you smaller sticky-blood spikes, eating slower and eating a smaller volume helps reduce the usual after-eating spikes. You've heard the admonitions "mindless eating" and "your eyes are bigger than your stomach." That's true – and inflammatory! Here's what science says about some practical food-serving tips to help you be satisfied with smaller amounts:

Serve food in smaller containers. Serving food in smaller bowls, smaller plates, smaller forks and spoons, and taller, skinnier glasses prompts people of all ages to eat less.

Out of sight, out of stomach. After you serve yourself, remove the large serving bowls from the dinner table. If you stare at the full bowl of pasta in front of you, you'll impulsively grab more. If you have to get up and find the bowl, even a few feet away, you're likely to eat more slowly and less. When you have to get up and walk to your next serving, you tend to eat less.

Do an experiment. Try this anti-inflammatory eating experiment: Prepare the same dinner for two evenings. One night eat it in a quiet and romantic place in your home with candlelight, soft music, and next to a window. The next night eat dinner at a well-lit, cluttered, noisier kitchen table. Because our gut brain and head brain are more in tune with each other, you are more likely to eat less and dine longer in the more relaxed setting.

Think Before You Eat

You may have heard this behavioral advice: think before you act. Here's a piece of similar nutritional advice: think before you *eat*. Before

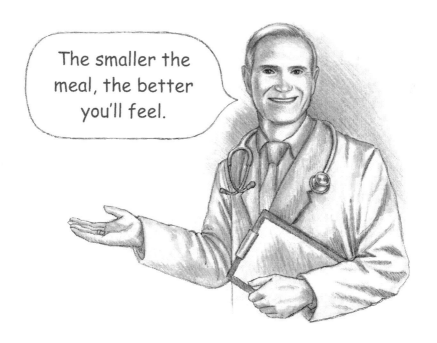

you give in to a craving that is likely to harm your health, say sitting in front of a TV and downing a donut, imagine the "donut effect" on your body. Imagine what the food is going to do to you before you eat it: sticky stuff sticking on the tissues of your brain, blood vessels, gut, and joints. Every time you see a donut, or even think of eating one, let the sticky thoughts trigger sickly images. This *negative conditioning* eventually programs your brain to reject donuts instead of crave them.

SPIKE-LESS SUPERFOODS

Spike-less foods	Spike-more foods
• Seafood	• Sweetened beverages (especially on an empty stomach)
• Legumes	
• Vegetables	• White bread
• Greens	• Overcooked pasta (see page 132)
• Plain yogurt	
• Nuts (especially walnuts)	• Big burgers
	• Fries
	• High-fructose corn syrup
	• Artificial sweeteners

My "salmon effect" story. I wasn't always fond of seafood but I was even less fond of getting inflamed with "-itis" illnesses. So when I saw a fillet of salmon I would imagine the omega-3 oils being good for my brain, eyes, heart, and joints, the vitamin D strengthening my bones and immune system, the astaxanthin being an anti-rust antioxidant, and so on. Eventually this *positive conditioning* clicked in and my brain convinced my body to crave salmon.

Remember, the head brain and gut brain are partners in inflammation health. Get them talking to each other. You can do that!

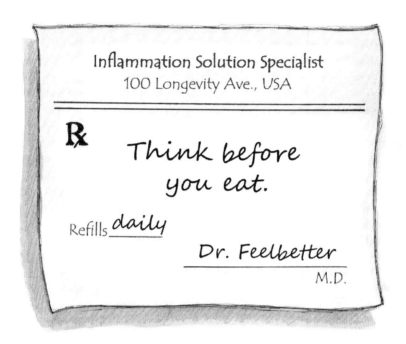

3. EAT SALADS FIRST

Salads are a healthy start to any full meal. When you eat a big green salad, two inflammation-balancing effects happen. The first is that you tend to eat less of the more "sticky" foods in the rest of the meal. The second is that by slowing the absorption of sugars and fats, the fiber in salads lower sticky spikes of inflamers during the entire meal. (See more about how salads blunt spikes, page 66.)

4. EAT MORE SEAFOOD AND LESS MEAT

As you learned from George's steak saga and Gracie's salmon tale, eating the same amount of seafood versus meat not only causes less postprandial lipemia (sticky stuff in the blood and slowing of blood flow), but seafood is a high-satiety food, helping you feel comfortably fuller while eating less. This is why successful weight-control programs add high levels of omega-3 fats to the diet. The healthy fat profile in seafood, especially wild salmon, enjoys a perk called *postprandial satiety*, meaning you get comfortably fuller sooner, so that fish-eaters are better able to curb overeating. (See more about the anti-sticky stuff effects of seafood, page 46, and the sticky effects of meat, page 132.)

Next time you're supermarket shopping, stare at a steak. Notice the meat is marbled and coated with white "sticky stuff". That's the result of all those sticky-carb grains used to fatten up the beef to weigh more and be worth more at market. Do you want your tissues to be streaked with sticky stuff, like the poor animal that sat around and ate junk food all day, or do you want them to be smooth and flexible like the swimming, real-food-eating salmon?

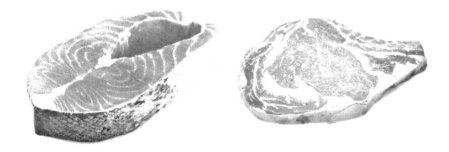

Salmon vs. Sirloin

5. ADD VEGETABLES TO YOUR MAIN COURSE

Instead of "fries," request a bunch of lightly steamed broccoli. Pairing other foods, especially meats, with vegetables somewhat reduces the postprandial lipemia (lowers sticky-stuff spikes).

6. DRINK UP TO LOWER STICKY STUFF

Here are drinks that are not only good to your gut, but good for your inflammation balance.

MY MEDICINE MEAL

I've enjoyed five trips to Japan to speak at scientific meetings on health and nutrition. During one of the trips, our Japanese host announced, "We're going to take you and Martha out for a medicine meal before your lecture." While I seldom eat a large meal before giving a talk, it would have been rude to refuse. The "medicine meal" was eight small courses of seafood, sea plants, and vegetables. After the meal I felt comfortably satisfied, neither too full nor hungry, but just right. Both my "gut brain" and my head brain were feeling good. Best talk I ever gave. Another good gut experience I noticed after dining on a "traditional Japanese dinner" (a 3-hour gastric delight of grazing on 15 courses of small portions interspersed with laughter and camaraderie) was that even though I ate a lot, I felt good, just the opposite of those bloated, blah, bad gut feelings that I would experience after gorging on an American buffet. It's amazing how the internal language of your gut says, "You feed me right, and you'll feel right."

Green Tea is a Good Anti-Inflammatory

I enjoy the anti-inflammatory effect of my daily cup of green tea. Why is green tea so great? The anti-inflammatory ingredient in green tea is EGCG. Cardiologists particularly like green tea because it naturally lowers lipids. Green tea seems to reduce the absorption of cholesterol, and it reduces the mischief that happens to dietary cholesterol by making the oxidized molecules less sticky. Among its many other health benefits, green tea reduces the blood levels of excess sticky blood fats, especially oxidized LDL. Neurologists call green tea a "neuroprotectant" because it helps remove amyloid (sticky stuff) deposits in the brain and, at least in experimental animals, helps grow new brain tissue. A healthful benefit of green tea is it diminishes the sticky-stuff spikes in the blood after eating a high-fat meal. Some of these effects occurred in drinking as little as two cups of green tea a day.

Why Wine Might Help Inflammation Balance

What would a health book be without wine, or an anti-inflammatory diet without this ancient remedy that has been perceived for centuries

DON'T DRINK SWEETENED BEVERAGES ON AN EMPTY STOMACH

To avoid sudden sticky-sugar spikes, if you absolutely must have that cola, sip it *slowly with your meal*. Think: real food tames the inflaming effects of fake food. Also, don't do diet drinks, as the artificial sweeteners can prompt the brain to crave carbs for hours after you've downed that "low calorie" drink containing neurotoxins.

as a health drink? Much to wine-lovers' delight, a glass of wine a day may help keep the "-itis" doctor away. Here are some wine-tasting tips to get the most healthful benefits from that Cabernet:

- **Respect your resveratrol.** The fermenting of red grapes produces a potent antioxidant in the polyphenol class called resveratrol. Wine researchers believe that this natural antioxidant may help reduce the effects of those sticky fats when sipped with a sticky meal, such as a grilled steak. While there are many other health claims to resveratrol, such as "the longevity factor in red wine" (including boosting immunity, lessening the stickiness of blood, and acting as a natural anti-coagulant), most of these studies were done in animals and test tubes, and with such high doses that you would have to drink a barrel of wine to get the same resveratrol effect as the studies showed.

- **Sip slowly.** Sip one glass (females) or two glasses (males) *slowly* and always with a full meal, never on an empty stomach.

- **Search the label for sulfites.** While sulfites may seem harmless to most people, some are highly allergic to them. They are used as chemical preservatives and are thought to act like an antioxidant within the wine. Also, the tannins, a natural biochemical byproduct of the fermentation process, may sometimes provoke a histamine-allergic response or migraine headaches.

The science of the anti-inflammatory effects of red wine is not solid enough to recommend that you start drinking wine if you don't already drink it.

7. DON'T OVERCOOK YOUR FOOD AND YOURSELF

In my pre-colon cancer days, I ordered a steak or burger with a nice crispy char. Overcooking your food overcooks – inflames – your body. Aging and inflammation have similar effects as when you overcook food. Meat and fish are the biggest examples. While people who eat the most fish have the fewest heart attacks, the more fried fish a person eats, the higher their risk of heart attacks. Aging of the tissues, especially the skin, depends on how you care for it. People who age too fast have subjected themselves to the same biochemical aging that happens to overcooked food – they overcooked their tissues with too much sticky stuff. The sticky food chemicals that stick to your tissues are called AGEs (see page 45) and are also known by the unappetizing term *glycotoxins*.

Glycation is a chemical process that makes otherwise healthful biochemicals in food sticky and unhealthful in your body. One of these is LDL cholesterol. Persons who eat the most overcooked or fried foods tend to have the highest level of glycated or sticky LDL. The reason animal-based foods, especially red meats, form the most AGEs, or very sticky stuff, is that these meats contain more of the type of fats that form sticky chemicals when they are overheated.

Careful cooking protects your body. Cooking with dry heat seems to be the worst. Cooking with moist heat, especially when the meat or fish is marinated or steamed, seems to be the healthiest because it produces less sticky stuff. Careful cooking yields a healthier meal. For example, cooking pasta *al dente* yields a tasty, chewy pasta with a lower glycemic index (the sugars are slower to release into the bloodstream and less sticky) than the sugar-rush, overcooked, mushy stuff typical in most American homes and restaurants. Overheating good oils, another example, causes a good fat to go bad.

One day I was explaining the "shuns" to a chef friend who got it right, "So over-inflamed means your body is overcooked."

Marinate meats. Stewing, poaching, or steaming is the healthiest way to cook meats and fish. Marinating in olive oil, apple cider vinegar, lemon juice, wines, and mustard garlic allows fewer AGEs to form. Try wet-sautéing (in half water, half oil). In plain chef talk, the more you grill your food, the more you're likely to grill your body. Next time you're grilling chicken or steak, imagine a similar process happening in the tissues of your body. When your body proteins are "cooked" with sugars, it's actually called "a browning effect," as happens when you grill your steak or chicken. Browning occurs when heated sugars and proteins react chemically with each other. The food turns brown and stiffens – it ages. The same stiffening happens in your body, especially in vulnerable tissues like arteries, eyes, and skin. Think stiff steak causing stiff arteries. If you must grill your food, at least marinate it, don't char it, and begin the meal with a big salad. (See how salads help tame inflammation, page 66.)

To motivate you to have burned your last burger, consider these cancer-causing facts: Over-grilling and charring forms carcinogenic compounds that even sound toxic: heterocyclicamines, glycoxals, and acrylamides. Shocking studies reveal that those who eat the most charred meats suffer the most breast, colon, and prostate cancers.

8. CARE ABOUT YOUR CARBS

Not only do fat spikes (hyperlipidemia) trigger sticky-stuff deposits in blood and tissues, sugar spikes (hyperglycemia) can be equally as sticky. Remember how you licked that brown, crusty stuff off the sugar-coated sticky bun you baked? Blood-sugar spikes bake the bake-able proteins in your blood and tissues, forming those sticky AGEs again. Chronic high blood sugar also glycates, or sticks to the normal

AVOID STICKY CHIPS

Americans consume the most chips and are the most inflamed. When starchy potatoes are fried at high temperatures, a sticky chemical, *acrylamide*, is formed.

Chips polluted with MSG are double trouble. MSG and its aliases (see list of anti-medicines, page 99) increase your cravings for more chips. Remember the ad, "Bet you can't eat just one!" Neurologists add another MSG caveat: You can actually develop an addiction to this neurotoxic chemical.

enzymes, such as superoxide dismutase, which are the body's natural clean-up antioxidants.

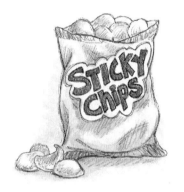

Besides just plain wearing out the overactive insulin-producing cells in the pancreas, another way chronically high blood sugar leads to type II diabetes is by damaging the cells due to the accumulation of sticky stuff, or inflammation. Yes, the epidemic of type II diabetes is just another in the long list of "-itis" illnesses caused by the simple saying: "You put sticky stuff in your mouth, you get sticky stuff in your tissues."

There are two camps when it comes to saying which foods cause the greatest sticky stuff effect: fats or carbs. Because it's most supported by science, I belong to the carb camp. Once American eaters started believing in the low-fat diet fad, they got more inflamed. In fact, many doctors have concluded that the biggest cause of the fattening – and inflaming – of Americans is when fats in foods were replaced with carbs. When you take fat out of food, you lessen the taste appeal. To make fat-less food more tasty, the scientists add more carbs. This has economic advantages: junk carbs are cheaper than healthy fats. And because junk carbs are less filling than healthy fats, you tend to eat more and buy more because junk carbs cause you to crave more junk carbs. Junk carbs mess up your healthy-craving centers that prompt you to "slow down and stop eating, you've had enough."

Good carbs and bad carbs. Here's how I explain good carbs and junk carbs to kids. A good carb plays with one, two, or three friends: protein, fat, and fiber. The more friends it plays with, the healthier the carb. When you eat these carbs, the three friends hold hands with the carbs to slow their rush into the bloodstream, preventing the spikes of sticky stuff. These friends tell the carb to slow down the rush to get into the bloodstream. This allows the gut to digest it more slowly and the body's blood delivery channels to deliver it more slowly and completely.

These good carbs also go by other biochemical names such as "low glycemic index" or "low glycemic load" carbs. These glycemic (sugary) terms simply mean how fast and how high what you put into your mouth elevates the level of sticky stuff in your blood. The lower the glycemic index (GI), the lower the level of sticky stuff in your blood.

Spike-less eating. Instead of the confusing terms "high and low glycemic," let's call them "rush carbs" and "slow carbs." "Rush carbs" spike more and tend to make you hungry, so you eat more. After eating "slow carbs," which spike less, you're satisfied longer and tend to eat less. Another label for carbs is "combo carbs," which are the carbs that are partnered with other nutrients such as fat, protein, and fiber, which slow down the rush into the bloodstream. "Solo" carbs are the worst, meaning they have no friends or partners. Try this experiment. Take a tablespoon of jelly (a solo carb) and spread it on a piece of white bread (a rush carb) and eat it. Notice an hour later you're hungry again because it has little protein, fat, or fiber. Spread the same jelly on top of a tablespoon of peanut butter on a slice of whole wheat bread.

The jelly becomes a combo carb because it is now combined with protein, fat, and fiber, and you feel fuller longer.

Low glycemic index, or low sticky-stuff carbs, are the ones found in nature, especially vegetables, whole grains, and fruits – in that order. Vegetables tend to have the lowest glycemic index because they enjoy two perks: they are high in fiber, which blunts the sticky-stuff effect, and they require longer chewing, which uses up a few more calories and gives you a more steady release of sugar into your bloodstream, allowing the body to use it almost as fast as you eat it. Whole grains also have this fiber effect, especially when partnered with protein. Fruits have the fiber effect, yet they don't have the sugar-blunting effect of protein and fat, which is why fruits are best consumed with meals that are partnered with protein and fiber, such as in a smoothie, a salad, or as a sweet accompaniment to the meal.

"Low-fat" often means added chemical carbs. One of the worst chemical carbs is high fructose corn syrup, which spikes blood insulin levels higher than cane sugar does. Sodas are seriously solo carbs. Sweetened drinks contain only sugar or high fructose corn syrup – no protein, fiber, or fat. So sugar rushes into the bloodstream, causing high levels of sticky stuff in the walls of the blood vessels and throughout the tissues of your body. I believe that the overconsumption of junk carbs, especially sweetened drinks, has been the number one contributor to the epidemic of inflammatory diseases. The consumption of too many junk carbs plus too much sitting are the two main contributors to making Americans the most inflamed people on earth.

Seductive sweet drinks. Sweetened drinks, especially those loaded with high fructose corn syrup, not only give you a rush of sticky stuff, they also prompt you to "eat or drink more." Perhaps that's why fast-food joints offer a cola with the sticky-stuff meal – so you want to buy and eat more sticky stuff.

DR. BILL ADVISES:

The Sticky Meaning of Fast Foods

The term "fast foods" signals various unhealthful effects on the body. It usually means foods that quickly increase the level of sticky stuff in your blood. In the long run it predicts a faster trip to the hospital or heart surgery center, and a faster path to the Ds: disabilities, disease, and doctors. The opposite of fast and sticky is slow and stable. Especially when eating out, ask yourself how this food and way of eating will affect your sticky-stuff blood level. This *cognitive connection,* also known as the cephalic stage of eating, or "mind before mouth," helps you be mindful of the healthful or unhealthful effects on your body before you get a stomach full of them. "Think before you eat" is a valuable disease-sparing health tip. (For more "Think before you eat" tips, see page 117.)

---

9. PARTNER YOUR INDULGENCES WITH ANTI-STICKY STUFF FOODS

Suppose you're about to indulge in sticky foods at an all-you-can-eat buffet. Here's how to ease the sticky-stuff effect on your blood and tissues. Shortly before you dine, do some vigorous exercise, such as walk around the restaurant parking lot, and do some isometrics (see why and how, page 217). Begin the meal with a hunk of fish, or down 3-4 grams (3,000 – 4,000 mg) of an omega-3 supplement. Even better, if you can pre-plan your pig-out a few days before, take this high dose of omega supplements daily. Research has shown that exercise and high doses of omega-3 supplements reduce the postprandial lipemia following a high-fat meal. (See related sections: Add Vegetables to Your Main Course 129, and Eat Salads First, page 127.)

CHASE YOUR MEAL WITH CHOCOLATE

Can a few squares of chocolate a day chase the sticky stuff away? Possibly so. Several years into my anti-inflammatory way of eating, I started noticing the goal of all dietary changes: my tastes were changing – in a healthy direction. I had re-conditioned my cravings. I did this by first learning what nutrients are best for keeping the sticky stuff under control, and then convincing myself to eat food containing those nutrients whether I liked them or not. This mindset helped me go from "don't like" to "like" to "crave." This is the sequence I preach in my medical practice. I started craving nutrients that were good for my body and shunning nutrients that were bad. One of those cravings was dark chocolate. There are many health benefits in chocolate, especially the antioxidants in cocoa called flavenols, a nitric oxide producer which is a powerful antioxidant. Yet it made no sense to swallow a powerful antioxidant – cocoa – mixed with junk sugars, which were pro-oxidants. So I had a little taste conditioning to do, starting with 60 percent cocoa, and gradually over three months increasing to 80 percent. It's amazing how you can re-shape your tastes. If I had started immediately with the healthy 80 percent, I would have perceived it as too bitter and not sweet enough, and it would have dampened my cravings. Now I consider 60 percent too sweet and 80 percent just right.

Then, I noticed I started craving two squares of 80 percent dark cocoa chocolate after my biggest meal of the day, the evening (a problem I'm still trying to solve). I thought it was more psychological than physical to end my meal on a sweet note. Then I realized that basically the inner wisdom of my body was telling me to eat a hefty dose of antioxidants to lower the sticky-stuff effect of the meal.

Unhealthy cravings are part of a body being out of inflammation balance; healthy cravings are a sign that your body is achieving inflammation balance.

Inflammation tips for chocolate lovers:

- The higher the cocoa percentage the healthier the chocolate.
- Dark chocolate is healthier than milk or white chocolate.

CHASE YOUR MEAL WITH CHOCOLATE (CONT'D)

- Pure *cocoa powder* usually contains more flavonoids (antioxidants). Once the cocoa gets processed into other forms (like chocolate), the antioxidant value decreases.

"Dutch" chocolate, or "dutched," is a chemical process that removes many of the antioxidants. Pure, dark chocolate is better.

---

10. GIVE YOURSELF AN OIL CHANGE

Ever since my health crisis, I've been developing my personal health plan: "everything works and nothing hurts." For one of my books I consulted the world's experts in preventing illness and inflammation. These scientists combined had personally published over 1,800 scientific articles, so I knew I was getting great advice. I asked them what would be one of the top pieces of advice to give patients who are suffering from various "-itis" illnesses.

Their anti-inflammatory prescription: eat more omega-3 oils and less omega-6 oils.

Oil eating made simple. Remember what you learned on page 13. To have a body in balance, especially inflammation balance, your two immune system armies, the "fighters" and the "healers," need to be in balance. When the fighters (also known as pro-inflammatories) outnumber the healers (also known as anti-inflammatories), your body does not enjoy inflammation balance and you hurt. Omega-3 oils (especially fish oil) and olive oil feed the anti-inflammatory armies, or healers. Omega-6 oils (vegetable oils such as soy, corn, and safflower) feed the pro-inflammatory armies, or fighters. When you enjoy omega balance in your body, you're more likely to enjoy inflammation balance. The general feeling among inflammation scientists is that the optimal omega balance is around 2:1 omega-6/omega-3 oils. Yet, the SAD is too high in omega-6s and too low in omega-3s, often at a 10:1 to 20:1 ratio.

Over the past several decades, the gradual increase in the omega-6/omega-3 ratio of oil-eating has paralleled the increase in "-itis" illnesses, and many scientists believe there is a cause-and-effect relationship. It's important to remember that most omega-6 oils are healthy oils. It's the *excess consumption* of them that contributes to inflammation imbalance. Here's why the omega-6 / omega-3 imbalance causes inflammation imbalance. Your tissues thrive on both of these oils, using them as part of the structural component of the cell membranes. Within the cell membrane there are enzymes that take

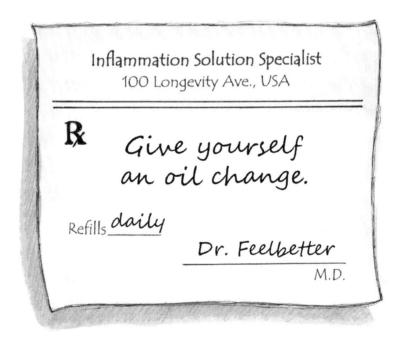

Inflammation Solution Specialist
100 Longevity Ave., USA

℞ Give yourself
an oil change.

Refills daily

Dr. Feelbetter
M.D.

YOUR OIL CHANGE GUIDE

Eat more	Eat less	Eat none
• Fish oil	• Corn oil	• Partially-hydrogenated oils
• Olive oil	• Soy oil	
• Flax oil	• Sunflower oil***	• Cottonseed oil****
• Nut oils*	• Safflower oil***	• Canola oil*****
• Coconut oil, virgin**		

*Nut oils, such as peanut, are excellent for cooking.

**Coconut oil has gotten an unscientific bad rap as a "saturated fat," but because of its healthy biochemical quirks, it doesn't behave like a saturated fat in the body and doesn't increase the sticky stuff in the blood vessels like the saturated fats in meats. Besides, new nutritional insights reveal that "saturated fat" isn't so unhealthful after all. Also, the MCT (medium-chain triglycerides) in coconut oil may improve cognitive function in patients with dementia, and are healthy fats for intestinal health.

*** The high oleic sunflower and safflower oils not only have a longer shelf life, but help lower the sticky blood fats.

****A cheap oil most likely to be contaminated with pesticides and contains one of the highest pro-inflammatory omega-6 / omega-3 ratios, greater than 200:1.

***** Too highly processed and chemicalized.

both omega-3 and omega-6 fats and, like bricklayers, assemble them into healthy cell membranes. When you eat an excess of omega-6s, the body uses up the available enzymes so there are not enough left over to utilize the omega-3s.

(For those who want a science-made-simple biochemical explanation of omega-6 and omega-3 oils, see my book *The Omega-3 Effect*, Little Brown 2012).

Remember, omega balance promotes inflammation balance.

11. EAT RAW VEGGIES — AGE SLOWER

Poor dental health can prompt us to chew our food less — just the opposite of what the rest of our gut would like us to do. Some older people tend to overcook vegetables to make them easier to chew, which tends to lessen the nutritional quality. Also, as we age, our digestive enzymes, which are natural chemical digesters, lessen, leading to indigestion. Let's start at the top end of our digestive tract, the mouth, to alleviate this downward spiral through the digestive tract. Besides keeping your teeth healthy, eating raw vegetables and fruits, which contain their own enzymes, helps with digestion. Raw foods release sugar in the gut more slowly than cooked foods since cooking breaks down some of the fibrous tissue that slows the absorption of the sugars. This is one reason why "instant" foods, such as oatmeal, have a higher sugar rush (higher glycemic index) than slow-cooked regular oatmeal. Also, the particle size of the food influences the glycemic load, or how fast the sugar gets into the bloodstream. The smaller the particle, the faster the sugar rush. "Instant" foods have smaller particle sizes, which is one of the reasons they cook faster and the reason they "cook" your body faster. Avoid "instant" foods. "Instant" means that the carbs go instantly into the bloodstream. Also, low-glycemic carbs, such as beans, keep you satisfied longer than high-glycemic carbs, such as potatoes.

12. EAT LESS, GET LESS INFLAMED

As we age, our natural fire-extinguishing system, or inflammation-balancing system, lessens a bit. The good news is that we have a built-in healing mechanism: as we age our resting metabolic rate (RMR), the normal level of metabolism from those millions of mini-fires that burn each minute throughout our body, naturally lessens because the natural burning of fuel from metabolism and repair lessens. We are programmed to eat less as we age because it seems our bodies need less fuel. Our bodies also may become more fuel-efficient as we age.

One way that our bodies become more efficient in using calories is that as we start to eat less, insulin sensitivity improves, so that our bodies have a better ability to regulate the right amount of insulin. Again, high insulin blood level is a sticky-stuff marker. Since insulin sensitivity often declines with increasing age, eating less helps slow this natural decline. Studies have also shown that eating less naturally lowers the level of one type of sticky stuff, the pro-inflammatory cytokine interleukin-6.

Here's what science says about the anti-inflammatory effects of eating less:

- Decreases levels of pro-inflammatory cytokines – sticky stuff.
- Increases brain-growth natural neurochemicals to improve cognitive function.
- Lessens neurodegenerative diseases.

Eating less is another diet-changing tool to lessen your chances of getting one of those neurodegenerative illnesses, such as Alzheimer's. Eating less is a prescription for neuroprotection.

CHAPTER 4

Move to Your Body's Content

Movement can heal your hurts. Suppose you did your homework and selected a top doctor for consultation to treat your "-itises". You say to Top Doc, "Doctor, I'm a show-me-the-science type of patient. I won't do anything to my body that is not backed up by solid science. I want the most scientifically-sound prescriptions to heal my hurts." Top Doc responds, "I'm also a show-me-the-science doctor. I won't prescribe any 'medicine' that is not backed up by science. So I'm going to give you the simplest, most scientific, and easiest prescription that

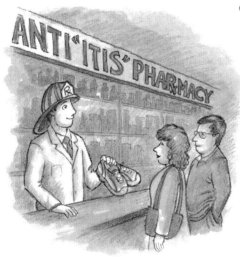

everyone can do." Top Doc scribbles on her prescription pad, "Move!" adding, "The more you move your sore joints, the less they will hurt."

You've heard of the "use it or lose it" advice that applies to most vital organs, especially the brain, heart, and muscles. The same is true of your joints. Your body is meant to move, especially your joints. Like the muscles, brain, heart, and bones, the more you use them the stronger they get. Movement moves your body into inflammation balance.

Move your body from hurting to healing. Mother's wisdom applies to all ages: "Go outside and play." The older we get, the less we move, and the more "-itis" illnesses we get. Any correlation? Yes. The epidemic of "sitting diseases" can be cured by one word: "Move!" Movement mobilizes your body's natural anti-inflammatory medicines. Remember, "-itis" illnesses means your body is out of biochemical balance. Movement helps put your body in balance.

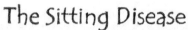

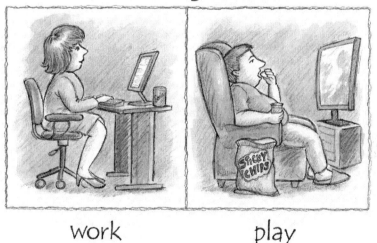

"How many hours a day do you sit?" may be the newest question your healthcare provider asks. The body is made to move. The more we sit, the more "-itises" we are likely to get. Because scientists are uncovering hidden therapeutic benefits to movement, there is a new label creeping into doctors' vocabulary – "sitting disease." Move more, sit less, hurt less. That's just what the "-itis" doctor ordered.

Besides suffering the inflammatory effects of our SAD, another SAD (sitting American disease) is inflaming us. Here are some SAD statistics: A 2010 Nielsen study revealed that the average adult watches 5.2 hours of television per day. Children average 8.2 hours a day sitting watching television or playing video games, leaving little time for play. A sick partner to the sitting disease is the *indoor disease*. (See Go Outside and Play, page 180.)

MOVING VS. SITTING: WHAT'S IN YOUR LIFE?

When you move you:

- Open your internal pharmacy (page 147).

- Squirt therapeutic oils into your joints (page 193).

- Make your own natural anti-inflammatories.

- Have a better back.

- Prevent Nature Deficit Disorder.

- Enjoy higher levels of "happy hormones".

- Have fewer "-itis" illnesses.

- Are more likely to stay happy.

- Enjoy longevity.

When you sit you:

- Internal pharmacy stays closed.

- Joints get sore.

- Back gets sore.

- You are more likely to get sick.

- You are more likely to get depressed.

- You are more likely to get inflamed.

- Diabetes, cardiovascular disease, arthritis, and Alzheimer's happen.

- You have a shorter lifespan.

When I was putting together my personal health plan (mainly to keep from getting "-itis" illnesses), I thought about how the human body is the greatest of all machines, the only one that is self-maintaining. Somewhere, I suspected, inside this magnificent machine is a giant internal medicine pharmacy that dispenses the right medicines to keep the body in inflammation balance. Wouldn't it make sense that your body could make its own anti-inflammatory medicines that are automatically dispensed at the right dose, at the right time, custom-made just for you so they'd have no side effects? That's exactly what can happen inside your body. And they're free! Your insurance plan will love you! Where in the world of your body's workings is this pharmacy and what medicines does it make? You will soon find out.

A NOBEL NIGHT TO REMEMBER

Eager to learn where in the body this personal pharmacy is located, and what anti-inflammatory medicines it makes, I invited to our home for dinner the scientist who would give me the answer, Dr. Lou Ignarro, who won the Nobel Prize for discovering the workings of this internal pharmacy. After our "salmon at sunset" dinner, I got out my notepad and the scientist began teaching the student.

Dr. Lou revealed that this pharmacy lies hidden in the endothelium, that one-cell layer that lines the blood vessels like pavement on a freeway. I was fascinated with this finding since most people don't know what the endothelium is or what it does. As Lou was teaching me about the endothelium, I thought of the term "the silver lining." Keeping your silver lining smooth gets my vote as a top path to health. Once upon a time the endothelium was thought to be nothing more than wallpaper lining the walls of the blood vessels. It was thought to be just a permeable layer of cells that nutrients squeak through to get from the bloodstream into the tissues. Thanks to Dr. Lou's research, now we know that the endothelium is the largest endocrine organ in the body. If you opened all the blood vessels and spread them out flat, the endothelium would cover a surface area of more than two tennis courts.

The cells of the endothelium are like closely-placed tiles on a countertop. But these tiles don't just sit there, they do something. The endothelium is like the chemical command center of the vascular system. It is your internal medicine doctor within, constantly sensing the medical needs of your body and responding to these needs by dispensing the right medicines, at the right dose, and at the right time.

As Lou, the scientist, was explaining to me, the student, in biochemical terms how these small molecules are proteins known as "biologically active" substances, I was sketching a simple line drawing that became the basis for the illustration on page 156.

"So, Lou, there are trillions of tiny medicine bottles within the endothelium. These bottles squirt natural anti-inflammatories into our bloodstream as needed?" Lou acknowledged that my medicine bottle analogy was scientifically correct and was a graphic way of explaining this internal pharmacy to novices. The key to health and inflammation balance is to keep the medicine bottles, your internal pharmacy, dispensing the natural anti-inflammatory medicines that you need when you need them.

One of the medicines in your pharmacy are natural anti-inflammatories, also called antioxidants, similar to the ones that are in richly colored fruits and vegetables. Think of the medicine bottles inside your endothelium as acting like trillions of tiny pharmacists. The better you feed and care for these pharmacists within, the more appropriate the medicines they dispense for you.

The better your blood flow, the better your health. One of the most overlooked and undervalued causes of poor health is poor blood flow to tissues. A medical truism: Each organ is only as healthy as the blood vessels that nourish it. This is why one of the top health effects of The Inflammation Solution Plan is keeping the lining of the blood vessels smooth, the walls of the blood vessels soft and flexible, and preventing sticky-stuff build-up inside the bloodstream.

ENDOTHELIALITIS

As we age, we not only wrinkle on the outside, but we wrinkle on the inside – the lining of our blood vessels. Here's an "-itis" you've never heard of, but it is the most prevalent and the most debilitating. *Endothelialitis* means an inflammation or "rusting" of the endothelium – the lining of the blood vessels. Because the health of every organ is dependent on the health of the blood vessels that nourish, protect, and repair each organ, this can become a total-body "-itis" illness. When sticky stuff, usually from two S's – sticky diet and sitting disease – sticks to the endothelium, the silver lining becomes a sticky lining. As a result of this inflammation, blood flow stalls and the release of natural endothelial medicines slows. This generally unknown "-itis" illness is one of the most serious ones, and the most preventable.

Blood vessel health depends upon:

- Flexible elastic walls that easily expand with each heartbeat. That's the pulse you feel.
- Little or no sticky stuff adhering to the lining of the blood vessels. (See what this does, page 18.)
- Less sticky stuff floating within the bloodstream, enabling the energy-carrying red blood cells to flow freely downstream to nourish the tissues.

A tale of two vessels. Gracie the Grazer, whom you met on page 120, is likely to enjoy smooth, stretchy vessels. Not so for George the Gorger (see page 121). After his meal the sticky stuff level in his blood is sky high. (Remember postprandial lipemia and postprandial glycemia, pages 43 and 121). His red blood cells stick together like congested cars on a highway, his vessel walls stiffen, and traffic slows.

This causes severe health problems to occur at both ends of the cardiovascular system:

Problems at the pump. George's heart muscle is forced to pump harder and faster to force the congested red blood cell traffic to move faster. The heart also has to pump stronger to increase the pressure outward against these stiff arterial walls (high blood pressure).

Problems downstream. As the heart pump is weakening at one end (congestive heart failure), tissues are starving downstream. A new term for this increasingly prevalent disease is hypoperfusion syndrome, which causes the following unhealthful effects: The tissues get underperfused from lack of enough blood flow, causing shrinkage of tissues that depend heavily on adequate blood flow, such as the brain. Sometimes these congested red blood cells just stop and clump together, causing a stroke or thrombosis. When the red blood cells stick together they can't worm their way into the tiny capillaries where the real transfer of nourishment occurs between the blood and the tissues. As the diagram on page 156 shows, each red blood cell is just a tiny bit smaller than the capillaries. This means that each red blood cell must be soft and flexible, allowing it to change configuration to work its way through the capillaries to get to the tissue cell where it's needed. Blood cells that are stiff and sticky get clogged up easily and never make it through the capillaries. Hence, the hypoperfusion syndrome. Translation: shrinking, hurting, dying tissues. In cardiology speak, the capillaries have lost their integrity.

Less blood flow equals shrinking brains. Until recently, the heart got all the attention as the organ most harmed by stiff and sticky blood vessels. Now, more researchers have turned their attention to the brain. Because it's such a hardworking and high metabolizing tissue, the brain requires a rich and steady blood flow, sort of like farmland needs lots of irrigation channels to grow the best produce. Recent insights into brain / blood flow dynamics reveal that stiff and sticky blood vessels may be one of the main underlying causes of neurodegenerative diseases of aging, such as Alzheimer's. To reflect this, a new term is appearing in the doctor's bag of diseases: *cerebral hypoperfusion syndrome.* Translation: Less blood flow, less mental acuity.

New technology providing windows into the brain have actually shown that middle-age people with high blood levels of sticky stuff and an excess waist size have shrinkage of the brain. The parallel between the blood vessels getting stiff and sticky and brain function getting slower is becoming more apparent. To support this suspicion, neuroimaging studies show hypoperfusion causes degeneration, mainly in those areas of high blood supply and in those areas associated with memory. In a nutshell, brain researchers conclude that the slower the blood flows to the brain, the slower the brain is able to think.

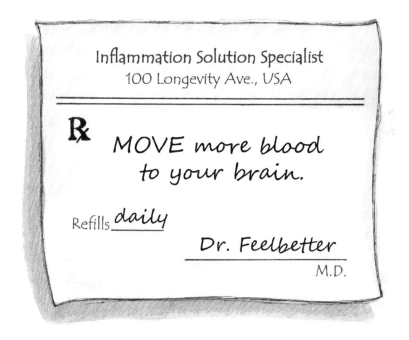

Inflammation Solution Specialist
100 Longevity Ave., USA

℞ MOVE more blood to your brain.

Refills *daily*

Dr. Feelbetter
M.D.

There are two ways to slow the usual cognitive impairment of aging and the cerebral hypoperfusion syndrome:

1. Stick to the six-S anti-inflammatory diet.

2. Move more!

When you move your body, you move more blood to the vital organs, especially the brain. In fact, studies have shown that movement increases *brain growth factor*, a natural brain growth fertilizer that helps your brain garden grow new crops, so to speak. Some fascinating studies show that regular brisk exercise increases brain volume, especially in those cognitive centers of the brain most affected in dementia and Alzheimer's.

HOW MOVEMENT MAKES YOUR NATURAL ANTI-INFLAMMATORY MEDICINES

My next question was, "Lou, how does a person open these medicine bottles to dispense the natural anti-inflammatories?"

Lou gave me a one-word answer to opening these medicine bottles – exercise – and that's the discovery that won him the Nobel Prize. The student in me keeps thinking that every time I talk to scientists, it comes back to what our mothers said decades ago, "The key to health is to eat your fruits and veggies and go outside and play."

He went on to explain what happens to your pharmacy when you walk fast, run, swim, dance, or do any brisk movement. The blood flows faster across those medicine bottles in your silver lining, your endothelium. The fast-moving blood fluid creates an energy field, called a *shear force*, which opens the medicine bottles to release the medicines you need.

Here's why I started nicknaming Lou "Dr. NO." I was mesmerized by finally having a scientific explanation for the doctor's advice to "exercise more." Lou got more biochemical: When you move, the blood flows faster across the endothelium, or the tops of the medicine bottles, producing a natural biochemical called nitric oxide, or NO. NO acts like a pharmacist that opens the medicine bottles and dispenses the medicines you need. The endothelium has its own antioxidant and anti-inflammatory properties to keep the silver lining healthy to make lots of NO. NO eats up free radicals so it decreases oxidative stress, or sticky stuff deposits, on your arteries. NO itself is an antioxidant and anti-inflammatory, which is why the endothelium is protective against arterial inflammation, sort of like self-resurfacing a well-traveled highway. This is how it protects against sticky stuff build-up, stroke, and heart attack. Exercise increases the production of circulating endothelial progenitor cells, self-repair cells for a damaged silver lining. Endothelial dysfunction is basically an inflammatory disease of the vessels. Aging is associated with endothelial dysfunction, which means the older we get the more we need to move.

How NO delivers more blood to needy tissues. Suppose you're running on a treadmill. Your moving muscles tell your heart, "I need more energy to work harder. Pump more blood faster." The faster the blood flows across the endothelium, the more NO it releases, which acts as a vasodilator, meaning it makes the blood vessels open wider so they can deliver more blood to the moving and hurting muscles. The next time you drive on a freeway, imagine your blood vessels are like a freeway. During rush-hour suppose the highway automatically widened into extra lanes so the traffic moves faster and doesn't clog up. This is what happens in your endothelium. When you move, your highways (blood vessels) widen and more blood flows to your muscles. In the case of inflammation of the muscles or joints, the more blood flow to those hurting tissues, the better they heal.

Have fun with your pharmacy story. Next time you're walking on a gym treadmill or with friends, shout, "Oh, it feels so good to be making my own medicines!" After the surprised looks subside, proceed to share your newly-found endothelial knowledge.

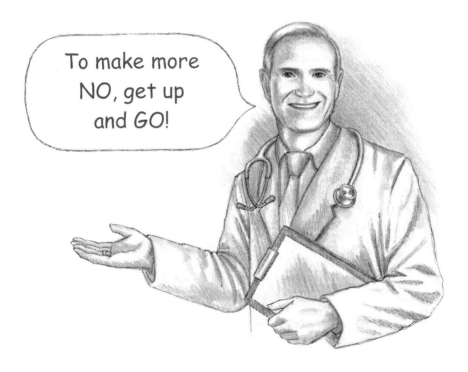

Keep your pharmacy open. Back to my sticky stuff explanation of "-itis" illnesses. In many people with "-itis" illnesses, their internal medicine pharmacy is closed because sticky stuff (often known as plaque) is deposited on the endothelium, keeping the medicine bottles from opening. This "-itis" illness is called *endothelial dysfunction* (see illustration, page 156.) When you exercise, the widened blood vessels send signals to those medicine bottles to dispense medicines that do all kinds of good healthful things for you, such as elevate your mood, keep the sticky plaque off the endothelium, and release natural anti-inflammatories to tame those "-itis" illnesses, and much more. In a nutshell, the more you move, the faster your blood flows, the wider your blood vessels are to nourish the hurting tissues, and the sticky stuff is kept off the lids of the medicine bottles so that your natural anti-inflammatories can be released when you need them.

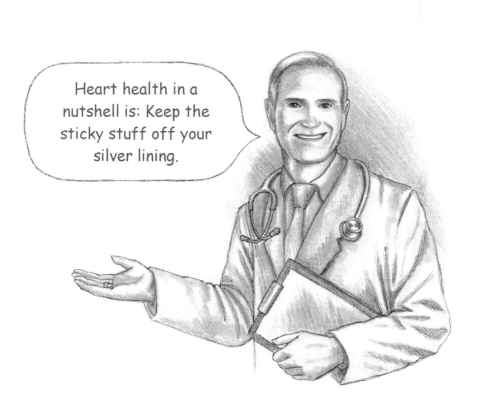

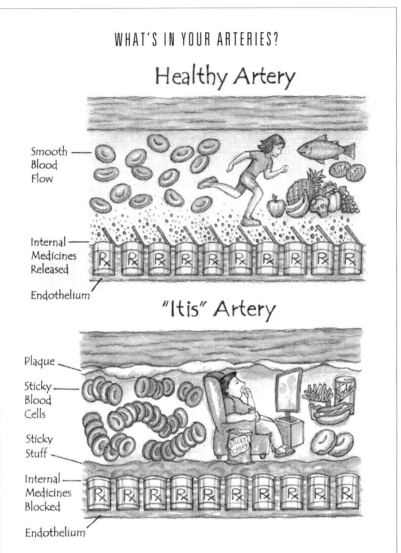

WHAT'S IN YOUR ARTERIES?

Healthy Artery

Smooth Blood Flow

Internal Medicines Released

Endothelium

"Itis" Artery

Plaque

Sticky Blood Cells

Sticky Stuff

Internal Medicines Blocked

Endothelium

The person who enjoys healthy arteries does the inflammation solution: eats anti-sticky stuff foods and supplements, grazes on healthy food, and moves a lot. This person's natural anti-inflammatory pharmacy is open 24/7 so she enjoys a "healthy bod." The "iBod" (a body full of inflammation) sits too much and eats too much sticky stuff. His pharmacy is closed.

This is why movers, more so than sitters, have smoother, softer, and larger coronary arteries. Also, people who move more have many more tiny blood vessels (capillaries) that nourish the tissues, sort of like building more irrigation channels to better nourish the soil. People who upgrade from sitters to movers often first notice healthier skin, because they have increased their nutrient irrigation to these tissues. That's why the age-old prescription for health is the dynamic duo, *diet* and *exercise*. Diet keeps the sticky stuff off the medicine bottles and exercise opens them up.

When Mr. Itis painfully walks into my office and says, "Doc, my joints are so sore, yet I'm afraid of the side effects of all those anti-inflammatories I have to take. Is there a safer medicine?" I prescribe, "Move!"

Another sticky stuff story. I continue to have fun with the sticky-stuff explanation of inflammation, perhaps because it's one of those concepts scientists have difficulty keeping simple and making fun. In June of 2013, I was invited to speak at a scientific meeting in Japan. I used the sticky-stuff analogy to try to explain inflammation of the endothelium, and it turned out to be one of the most memorable and popular topics of the day. It's challenging when you're talking to a scientific audience via an interpreter. As I was explaining the difference between the smooth silver lining of a healthy artery and the rough lining of an inflamed artery, I noticed the interpreter making very happy and very sad faces and the audience mimicking her. Since the speaker is at the mercy of the interpreter, and you're never quite sure if what you're saying and what the audience is hearing is the same, I enjoyed watching this facial language. The interpreter later explained that she used the river and riverbank analogy. When you put garbage into a river, the garbage sticks to the riverbank and you get *"doro doro,"* or a dirty river and dirty river bank. When there is no garbage in the river, you get clean water and a clean riverbank, or *"sera sera."* Which do you want in the rivers of your bloodstream: *"doro doro"* or *"sera sera?"*

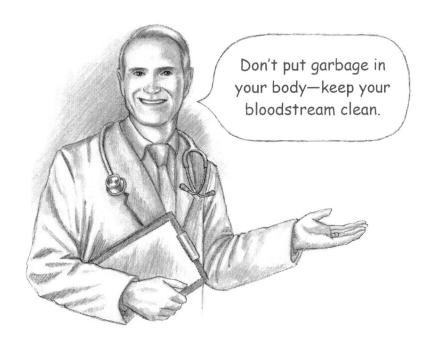

Don't put garbage in your body—keep your bloodstream clean.

Wired To Walk

It seems that the inflammation epidemic is a consequence of the sitting disease. Neurologist Eva Selhub, in her book, *Your Brain on Nature*, makes the compelling point that in human adaptation, man was designed to walk many miles a day for sheer survival. So when we walk our brains are naturally programmed to recognize that we are doing an activity that is worth doing, a lot. The theory of anthropologists is that walking filled the body and brain with health-promoting biochemicals to keep man walking to survive. Researchers have recently validated this "wired to walk" theory by discovering the healthful neurochemicals the body and brain makes while walking: natural antidepressants, brain growth neurochemicals, happy hormones, and anti-inflammatories.

So, we are wired to walk, not to sit. Here are the effects of consistent exercise on the body and brain:

- Increases telomere length. Telomeres are the ends of our chromosomes that shorten with aging.

- Regulates mood-modulating neurotransmitters. In fact, recent research reveals that exercise regulates serotonin production as do antidepressant drugs, but without the side effects.

- Increases the production of brain-derived nerve growth factors, which itself has antidepressant properties.

- Increases the growth of blood vessels to the brain, which increases blood flow to the brain. So not only does it increase beneficial neurochemicals, it increases the highways to deliver more of these neurochemicals.

- The older we are, the more we need to move. Movement stimulates the release of one of your body's top healing hormones, human growth hormone (HGH). This "more walking – more HGH" relationship becomes even more important as we age because HGH begins to drastically decrease in people over 50, especially in those who sit too much.

How Movement Lubricates and Heals Sore Joints

Moving your body helps heal sore joints by:

1. **Providing nourishing blood flow to your tissues.** As you learned earlier in this chapter, the more blood flow, the more healing nutrients get into those hurting tissues.

2. **Squirting more natural lubricants, called *synovial fluid*, into your joints.** In Chapter Seven you will learn how your joints make their own medicines when you move them.

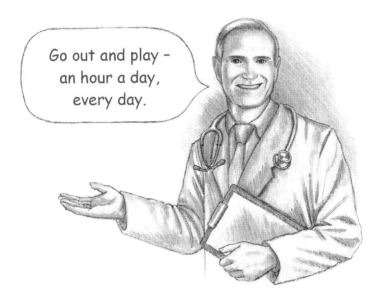

3. **Strengthening the tissues that support the joints.** The stronger you make your muscles and bones; the stronger these tissues support the joints. In doctor lingo, weakened muscle is called "disuse atrophy". Use it or lose it.

Knee, hip, shoulder and back pain top the "-itises" that lead most persons into the two Ds: disability and doctors' visits. In Chapter Seven, you will learn how to move the pain and stiffness out of your knees and other joints.

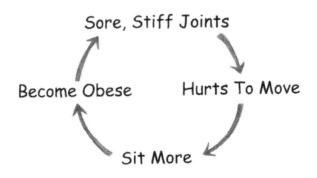

START LOW, GO SLOW

In untrained persons, a sudden bout of unaccustomed exercise can amp up the production of pro-inflammatory chemicals and free radicals. A Harvard study showed moderate exercise within one's own comfort zone is healthier. Exercise that is too strenuous, too long, and way above a person's comfort zone may increase oxidative stress (wear and tear on the muscles) and aggravate inflammation. In fit persons, especially when it becomes a consistent daily tonic, exercise has both antioxidant and anti-inflammatory effects.

As a person gets progressively more fit, the body adapts by upgrading its antioxidant and inflammation defenses so that exercise eventually helps put the body back into inflammation balance. This mechanism explains why the blood markers of chronic inflammation are lower in persons who are physically fit. This also explains why inflammatory markers are higher in sitters.

No burn, no earn! Expert fitness trainers no longer teach the "no pain, no gain" method. Exercising until you hurt can be unhealthy. Yet, if you are exercising to build muscle (see how building more muscle trims your waist, page 167) gradually increasing the weight and the duration of lifting until you feel the "burn" is a safe and effective way to exercise.

ANOTHER INFLAMMATION: ERECTILE DYSFUNCTION (ED)

Here's a sure fire way to get more men moving. You may have heard the best way to a man's heart is through his stomach. Really, a better way is through a more vascular organ. Most men who have problems with their penis (ED) also have problems with their heart (endothelial dysfunction). My friend, let's call him John, had an "-itis" body waiting to happen, but I just couldn't convince him to get off the couch and clean up his sticky diet. In fact, I opened our conversation with, "John, you're an *iBod*, a body riddled with inflammation." I showed John a diagram of what his arteries probably looked like. What's healthful for the heart is also perfect for the penis. The man-to-man talk progressed from endothelial dysfunction to ED. The next day he started consistently doing what his loving wife had advised, "Eat more fruits, vegetables, and seafood, and go outside and play."

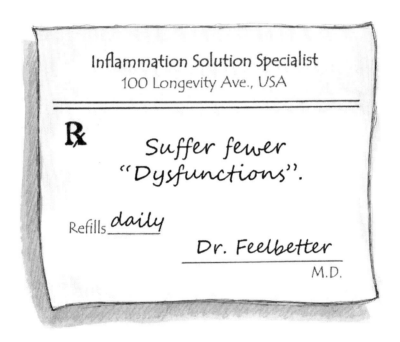

Inflammation Solution Specialist
100 Longevity Ave., USA

R Suffer fewer "Dysfunctions".

Refills daily

Dr. Feelbetter
M.D.

CHAPTER 5

Reduce Your Waist

"Bill, I have a bad back," Bob complained. "Bob, you have a bad back because you have a big belly," I answered. A leaner waist lessens inflammation. A big belly produces big inflammation. Suppose you were motivated to make only one change or have one goal to reduce your "-itis" illnesses. What change would you make or goal would you have? Or, suppose you consulted a Top Doc to heal your hurts. You open your consultation, "Doctor, I don't have a lot of free time, so just give me one change I can make to help heal my hurts." Top Doc complies, "I'm going to give you the most important goal you can set to heal your hurts: *reduce your waist*." Surprised, you wonder what your waist size has to do with your arthritis. Here's why shedding three to six inches off your belly size is one of the most important therapeutic ways to shed some of those "-itis" illnesses.

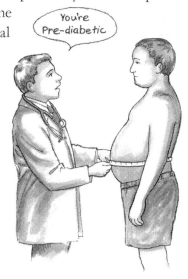

If your doctor dubs you "inflammation belly," the diagnosis is biochemically correct. To motivate the parents of my young patients to get and stay lean, a few years ago I stopped using the wimpy word "overweight." I upgraded this to a more biochemically-correct and life-changing label: "Joe, you're *pre-diabetic*."

Here's another SAD statistic: Doctors estimate that over fifty percent of Americans over age 50 may be pre-diabetic.

CLOSE YOUR INFLAMMATION FACTORY

The shape of your waist mirrors the shape of your inflammation balance. When a patient goes to a doctor for "-itis" counseling, if the physical examination merits it, the first measurement is waist size – which surprises many patients. Because of new insights about abdominal fat – dubbed "toxic waist" – more and more doctors are valuing waist size or waist-hip ratio as a very informative vital sign. In fact, your personal waist-o-meter, such as a skirt, belt, or pant size is more meaningful than your scale weight. Here's why.

Most fat cells, called adipocytes, are just storage sites for excess fat. They sit in your cheeks and thighs and get larger when you eat more than you burn and get smaller when you burn more energy than you eat. So do abdominal adipocytes, but they behave differently biochemically from the fat cells elsewhere in your body. They are basically a *chemical factory*, an actual organ that produces harmful biochemicals that contribute to cardiovascular disease, high blood pressure, mood disorders, diabetes, and cancer.

Excess abdominal fat is a chemical factory for cytokines – inflammatory biochemicals that, in excess, throw the body into inflammation imbalance. Another pro-inflammatory that excess belly fat cells dump into the system is the inflammatory chemical interleukin-6. Excess abdominal fat is one of the common reasons for inflammatory markers, such as CRP (see page 239), to be high.

Belly fat is a good news / bad news issue. The bad news is it's the easiest to put on. The good news is it's the easiest to take off. Excess abdominal fat is usually the first to go because of a biochemical quirk in those belly fat cells. They respond better to diet and exercise than does fat elsewhere in the body. Diet and exercise cause the fat in these cells to be converted to free fatty acids, which are then oxidized and burned as fuel. When fats are burned, these cells shrink.

How bellies get fat. A big belly literally throws your body out of balance – physically and biochemically. While the right percentage of body fat is healthful, excess *abdominal* fat has become so prevalent and so unhealthful that a big belly now has its own medical disease label: *abdominal adiposity.*

Unhealthful hormones. As the belly grows, it becomes an extra endocrine organ, and the hormones it pours into your body are not healthful. These unhealthful hormones, dubbed *adipokines*, behave in your body in just the opposite way your normal healthful hormones do. Remember our hormonal symphony explanation of wellness and inflammation balance (see page 14)? Your healthful hormones are the dials that regulate and balance your bodily functions, such as blood sugar, blood lipids, blood pressure, and blood stickiness (clotting).

The adipokines from the big-belly fat cells create harmful hormones that throw the body out of balance: high blood sugar, high blood lipids, and high blood pressure. "Fat scientists" (I mean those who study the medical effects of too much belly fat) have uncovered several dozens of these chemical crooks, the adipokines that rob the body of balance.

Learn about leptin. Leptin was discovered in 1995. To remember what leptin does, think of it as the **lean**est or eat-**less** hormone. Leptin (derived from the Greek word meaning "thin") is normally released from fat cells in the body and circulates into other cells where it removes excess fat deposits. For example, leptin gets into the cells of the pancreas and, by its own chemical language, says, "I'll get rid of the excess fat globs to make more room for the cells that make insulin so they can better do their job. I protect against insulin resistance or type II diabetes." So you may conclude that the more fat we have, the more leptin we make, and that is good. Wrong! Like any hormone, when the body makes too much of it – when the leptin dials are too high – the body, in its wisdom, fights against the excess or "becomes resistant" to leptin. A new disease has been added to the already overweight list of modern man-made diseases: *leptin-resistance*. Like *insulin resistance*, this is another case of a good hormone gone bad. When we let our body get out of physical balance, it gets out of biochemical balance. In some persons, the excess leptin becomes a mutant. Instead of helping keep the body in inflammation balance, it increases the circulating level of inflamers – more sticky stuff, and throws the body into inflammation imbalance.

CARE ABOUT YOUR CALORIES

Caring about the *kind* of calories is much more important than *counting* them. Calorie-counting diets are not necessarily anti-inflammatory. Calorie-caring diets are anti-inflammatory. For example, suppose one person guzzles a 150-calorie cola, the junk carbs rush into the bloodstream as sticky carbs, many of which land in the belly as excess flab. Another person eats 150 calories, but in a salad. Two healthful perks happen: Many calories are used up just chewing and digesting the fiber-filled carbs and protein, and there are no sticky spikes.

Young Fat Cells Get Fatter

Leanness is especially healthful in the young, whose immune system is still maturing, and in seniors whose immune system is weakening. An over fat child is at high risk of becoming an over fat – and over inflamed – adult. An obese child is weighed down by an increased *number* of fat cells, or adipocytes, which is more difficult to lower than just shrinking the *size* of the excess fat cells like adults can do.

Another link between leanness and longevity has been discovered in that vital organ that, until reading this book, you probably knew little about – the endothelium (see page 19). Those extra belly fat sticky biochemicals travel around and in blood vessels and produce a very sticky inflammatory molecule called tumor necrosis factor (TNF-alpha), which blunts the NO effects of relaxing arteries. An unrelaxed or constricted artery leads to high blood pressure.

But the good news is when you lose this extra fat the sticky-stuff effect on your blood vessels lessens. Your sticky stuff can get less sticky. The Health ABC study (Health, Aging, and Body Composition) revealed that, not surprisingly, as the blood levels of sticky stuff (inflammatory markers CRP, IL-6, adhesion molecules and TNF) came down, so did the incidence of coronary artery disease. The researchers concluded that sustained weight loss is a safe and effective way to lower sticky-stuff levels in the blood.

YOUR "WEIGHT" IS NOT AS IMPORTANT AS YOUR WAIST

The new science of weight management – better called *waist* management – reveals that *body composition* influences inflammation health more so than scale weight. Say two persons each weigh 150 lbs. One has a body composition of toned muscle and 15 percent body fat. The other person weighs the same but has 25 percent of his body weight as fat, mostly around the middle. You guessed it! The higher-body-fat person is more likely to be an inflamed person.

To Reduce Your *Waist,* Reduce Your Waste

Excess belly fat behaves like dumping inflammatory biochemicals – sticky stuff – into your bloodstream. So shedding excess belly fat is another way to lessen the sticky stuff pouring into your tissues.

One evening after my lecture on how a big belly and big behind causes big "-itis" illnesses, a comedian in the audience summed it up: "To get the butt you want, move the butt you have!"

THE BIGGER YOUR BELLY, THE SMALLER YOUR BRAIN

Excess belly fat inflames and withers the brain by two mechanisms: it causes insulin resistance and high blood sugar, which inflames the brain; and it also spews out inflammatory chemicals that damage brain tissue. A study comparing the waist-to-hip ratios to measured structural changes in their brains found that persons with bigger bellies tended to have a smaller memory center, the hippocampus, which is often the first cerebral organ to shrink with dementia and Alzheimer's disease. Neurologists are beginning to find that, in general, the bigger the belly the smaller the brain tissue.

TAKE THE LOAD OFF YOUR JOINTS

Besides worsening "-itises" everywhere in your body, excess belly fat is particularly harmful to the knees and hips – those joints that bear the weight and wear and tear of a big belly. For every extra pound of excess weight you lug around, especially in the middle, that's 3-4 pounds of excess weight your knees have to bear. Also, watch a person with a big belly "waddle walk." Their hip joints and knee joints are so out of balance that every step they take causes excess wear and tear on these joints. In doctor talk, a person with a big belly and resultant waddle walk is a knee and hip replacement waiting to happen. According to orthopedic neurologist Dr. Vincent Fortanasce, for every fifteen pounds of excess weight you lose, you cut your chances of degenerative knee problems in half.

Resources for Waist Management: See the L.E.A.N. Anti-Inflammation Prescription

Our L.E.A.N. Program is time-tested and has proven tools to optimize your weight *and your health*. Both of these are our goals because not all programs are healthy and some can even cause you to be skinny but sick. Learn more about the L.E.A.N. program at DrSearsWellnessInstitute.org.

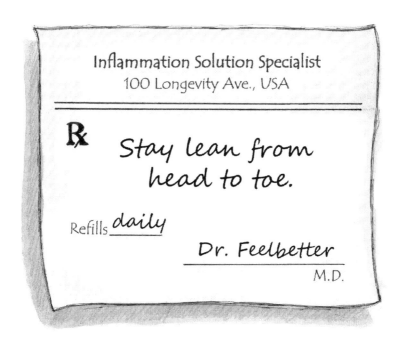

CHAPTER 6

Don't Worry, Be Less Inflamed

Yes, you can worry yourself sick. Yes, you can un-worry yourself well. Chronic, unresolved stress depresses the immune system. Oftentimes I hear, "My arthritis flares up when I'm stressed." Again, it's a question of balance. Some stress, like inflammation, is good; too much is bad.

HOW STRESS MAKES YOU SICK

Stress itself doesn't cause inflammation. It's how you handle it that counts. Your body has two dials for a stress response: one dial (called the sympathetic nervous system or SNS) turns up the level of circulating hormones when your body needs extra energy and needs to make quick decisions for its wellbeing. Suppose you need to run from a building on fire. Your SNS dials up extra biochemical turn-ons (stress hormones like adrenaline and cortisol) that increase your heart rate to pump more blood to your fast-moving muscles and blood-sugar fuel to your brain to make quicker decisions. Then, after the danger has passed, another dial (the parasympathetic nervous system or PNS) turns down the SNS and puts your body back in biochemical balance. When your body is in normal *stress balance*, the PNS and SNS

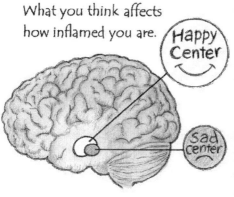

What you think affects how inflamed you are.

Happy hormones
blood pressure just right
heart rate just right
heart and brain stay healthy
fewer "itis" illnesses

Sad (stress) hormones
blood pressure too high
heart rate too fast
heart & brain wear out sooner
more "itis" illnesses

are in balance. When your body is out of stress balance, you dial up the SNS too high and the PNS too low.

Worry worsens all "-itis" illnesses in two ways. Chronic, unresolved stress weakens the immune system causing "-itis" flare-ups, and stress *increases your sensitivity* to pain. So, as you worry more, you hurt more.

The hormonal harmony (wellness) of the body means all these dials are interconnected and they monitor each other to behave. Suppose you keep your stress dial turned up and flood your body and brain with high stress hormone levels, especially cortisol. This also turns up your pro-inflammatory dial, putting your body into inflammation imbalance. Besides the direct effect of stress hormones, namely cortisol, being too high for too long, this imbalance results in chronically elevated blood sugar, which leads to increased AGEs and elevated blood insulin levels, which also stimulate increased levels of pro-inflammatory chemicals. To make the tissues even more sticky and inflamed, continued high levels of stress hormones render cells less sensitive to insulin, eventually increasing the risk of type II diabetes.

Because this normal dial-down mechanism weakens as we age, it takes longer for the elevated stress hormone to go back to baseline after a stressor. Because of this quirky mechanism causing stress hormones to be higher as we age, the older we get the calmer we need to be. Here's how chronic, unresolved stress inflames your vital body parts.

HOW STRESS MAKES YOU FAT

When we're stressed, we don't try to grab a bite of salmon. We typically reach for the nearest, sweetest stuff. The adrenaline rush and high cortisol stress response makes you hungry for carbs. (Remember, "stressed" spelled backwards is "desserts".) This is a similar mechanism to how stress can make you fat. Prolonged, high stress

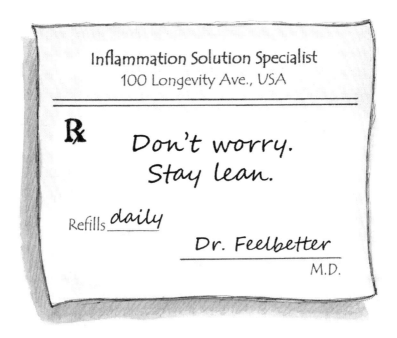

hormones, especially cortisol, prolong high levels of insulin, the fat-storage hormone. The stressful cycle is: high stress produces high insulin, which produces high fat, which produces more high insulin. Also, when you're stressed, your natural appetite-control center doesn't work well.

HOW STRESS IS HARD ON YOUR HEART

Remember, lessening inflammatory wear and tear on the lining of your blood vessels, naturally, is the prime goal of *The Inflammation Solution*, because your vital organs rely on healthy blood vessels to nourish them. Chronic, unresolved stress is a double whammy. Increased stress hormones cause prolonged high blood pressure (make blood vessels stiff) and dump sticky stuff (AGEs) on the endothelium. Using our highway health analogy, the higher the pressure of the blood flow through the vessels, the higher the force it exerts on the lining, like heavy trucks exert more wear and tear on a road and can spill more sticky tar on it. Then, to add more insult to injury, the inflammatory response interprets this as a mess and mobilizes its repair crew to fix it. The problem is it's often over-repaired, leading to more build-up and clots.

Chronic, unresolved stress also makes blood cells, especially platelets, more sticky and likely to clump together, which causes a cascade of more sticky stuff in your blood sticking to the sticky stuff that's already on the lining of your blood vessels. Chronic stress does a number on your coronary arteries. Normally, arteries dilate in response to an acute stress saying, "We need more blood to fuel those hardworking muscles." Yet during chronic stress, they actually narrow. An uptight mind gives you uptight blood vessels. Relaxing your mind relaxes your blood vessels.

One way stress triggers inflammation is by increasing the blood pressure. There is increased pounding against areas of increased turbulence and pressure in the arteries, like chipping potholes in a road that is overly traveled. This sets up the inflammatory response, which tries to repair – or over-repair – the potholes. More sticky stuff builds up, such as oxidized LDL, or sticky LDL. Eventually these blood vessels exposed to high pressure get so much sticky stuff in the lining and hard stuff in the walls (hardening of the artery) that they don't dilate or open up when traffic increases, like our analogy of the freeway automatically opening up by adding a few extra lanes during rush-hour. Now you have stiff vessels with sticky stuff running through them, and whatever is downstream doesn't get enough nutrients, and the organs start to get weak and tired. Cardiologists dub this scenario a "neurotic heart."

HOW STRESS BOTHERS YOUR BRAIN

Ever wonder why your "-itises" get worse when your mind gets stressed? The neurochemicals that regulate moods, such as the happy hormones serotonin and dopamine, are connected to the dials that balance inflammation biochemicals. So when your mood dials are out of balance (too high, anxiety; too low, depression), your inflammation control is also out of balance. Countless times I've heard friends say, "When my mind feels better, so do my joints."

When your mind hurts, so does your body. An uncomfortable fact of "-itis" life is that a person's perception of pain is amplified during depression.

There's a new word in the doctor's list of modern diseases: *neuroinflammation*. A startling statistic is that in 2013, neurodegenerative diseases (Alzheimer's, Parkinson's, multiple sclerosis) have overcome cardiovascular diseases as the top illness in America. The brain is now

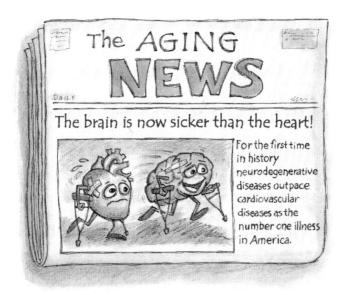

sicker than the heart. And yet, because a healthy brain needs healthy blood vessels, the two organs are partners in health – or illness. Why has the brain out-inflamed the heart as the main organ attacked by inflammation?

- The brain is 60 percent fat, which is why we are truly "fatheads." Fat is the tissue most vulnerable to damage by oxidation and inflammation.

- The brain (including the eye, which is really part of the brain) is the hardest working organ in the body. It uses at least 20 percent of all the food energy we eat, so it generates a lot of oxidative stress – sticky stuff.

- Brain tissue doesn't repair and regrow as fast as other tissues.

- Unlike the lungs, kidneys, and knee joints, we have only one brain.

- The hippocampus, the area of attention and concentration, emotional content, and memory is the area most attacked by

Alzheimer's. The hippocampus is the most vulnerable area of the brain because it has the most highly metabolized cells, needing the most blood supply and energy. Therefore, it is the most vulnerable and needs the most antioxidant and anti-inflammatory protection. Two NIH studies showed that three months of severe, unresolved stress could reduce the volume of the hippocampus by 14-20 percent.

Some neuroscientists even conclude that anti-anxiety and antidepressant medicines may work as anti-inflammatories, similar to what cardiologists are concluding about the mechanism action of statin medications.

Building your personal toolbox of stressbusters and discussing all the psychotherapy of stress management is beyond the scope of this book, yet there are some starter tools.

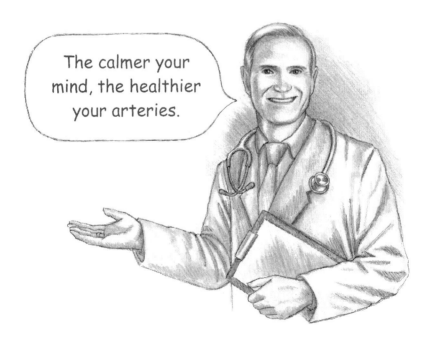

The calmer your mind, the healthier your arteries.

CHANGE YOUR MIND, CHANGE YOUR INFLAMMATION

Mind over inflammation. People who show more positive and less negative emotions often show a lessening of their "-itis" illnesses. Happy, positive moods dial up happy hormones, which dial down inflammation-aggravating biochemicals; chronic sad, negative moods do the reverse. Also, as we age we need a better stressbusting toolbox. Why? Because our normal stress hormone secretions don't dial down as quickly as we age. Circulating, resting blood levels of stress hormones, such as adrenaline and cortisol, tend to stay higher as we age. This stress effect on the brain even has a name: *glucocorticoid neurotoxicity*. Sounds like something you don't want to get!

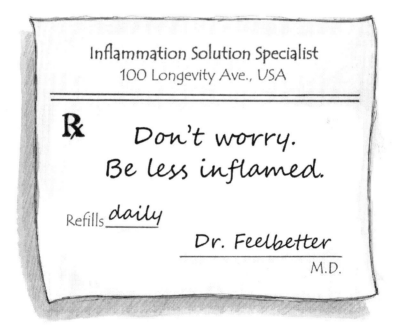

HOW STRESS CAUSES A PAIN IN THE GUT

I love how renowned stress neuroscientist Dr. Robert Sapolsky in his classic book, *Why Zebras Don't Get Ulcers,* describes digestion as "breaking down chunks of animals and vegetables so they can be transformed into chunks of human." While somewhat unappetizing, it is chemically correct. Besides the brain and heart, for some people the gut is the organ most bothered by chronic stress. There are several reasons for this. At least 70 percent of your immune system resides in the gut. Around 90 percent of the "happy hormone," serotonin, is made in the gut. Stress slows digestion. Starting at the top end, it decreases saliva secretion; giving you dry mouth and depriving the food you just ate of digestive enzymes (strike one).

Next, the otherwise vigorously contracting stomach slows down and stops mashing the food and secreting digestive enzymes, and the rest of your intestines slows down its snake-like dance (strike two).

Stress shunts blood flow from the gut to other organs. Because the body mistakenly believes you need these stress hormones to pump up your heart and muscles to always be on "high alert" even when you don't need to be, it diverts blood flow from your gut to help you survive. Stress interferes with the natural acid balance, which is why it's common to get more digestive problems, such as heartburn or reflux, during stressful times. In fact, many of the gastrointestinal upsets that fill doctors' offices – irritable bowel syndrome and "-itises" – are made worse by high levels of unresolved stress (strike three).

HOW STRESS CAUSES INFLAMMATION IMBALANCE

Again, that health word *balance.* Your stress response and your immune system have a similar balancing act for the health of your body. During a stressful response, say running out of a building on fire, your body dials up stress hormones to enable you to get out of the building. These stress hormones also dial up your inflammation fighters in case you need a higher level of protection against infection during that time. A healthy stress response system is meant to be quickly dialed up and then dialed down. If, however, your stress hormones stay dialed up, as in chronic unresolved stress, your immune system's inflammation army also stays on high-alert attack mode, leading to inflammation "-itis" illnesses (over attacks) and autoimmune diseases (self-attacks). Simply put, chronic stress not only weakens your natural immune army inside so you get sick more often, it causes your immune army to mistakenly attack its own soldiers — your tissues.

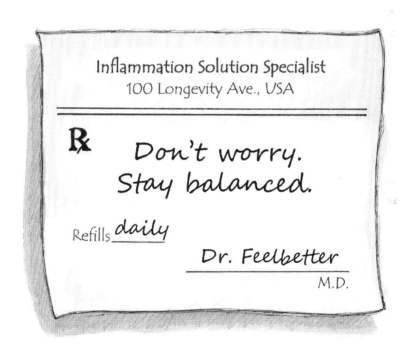

Inflammation Solution Specialist
100 Longevity Ave., USA

R Don't worry.
Stay balanced.

Refills daily

Dr. Feelbetter
M.D.

MY SIX FAVORITE STRESSBUSTERS

1. Go Outside and Play

Remember mom's medicine for boredom and bad behavior? "Go outside and play!" An exciting field of research, called the neuroscience of nature, proves that Dr. Mom was right. Enjoying the health effects of a walk in the woods or playing in the park is especially therapeutic in this modern age of windowless work cubicles and the artificial light of computer screens.

Neuroscientist and author of *Your Brain on Nature*, Eva Selhub, M.D., reveals exciting new science on how we are wired to walk through the giant "pharmacy of nature": woods, parks, beaches, mountains, oceans, and lakes. Movement balances the inflammation system. Moving in nature is even better medicine. The epidemic of "-itis" illnesses seems to have increased with the increase in the amount of time humans spend indoors. Any correlation? In my medical practice, I call it "The Indoor Disease", or another "D", Nature Deficit Disorder.

Here's a summary of what science says about nature being a powerful healer and anti-inflammatory:

- Dials down stress and inflammation hormones: mellows moods.
- Dials up relaxation and inflammation-balancing hormones. Increases serotonin.
- Calms brain and heart: decreases heart rate and high blood pressure.
- Stimulates an area in the brain that is rich in natural pain relieving opiates (shown by brain-imaging studies).
- Boosts immune system's NK cells.

- **A room with a view.** Some hospitals wheel patients outside into an atrium, and try to face the bed toward a window. Japanese studies show hospitalized patients whose beds face the window heal faster.

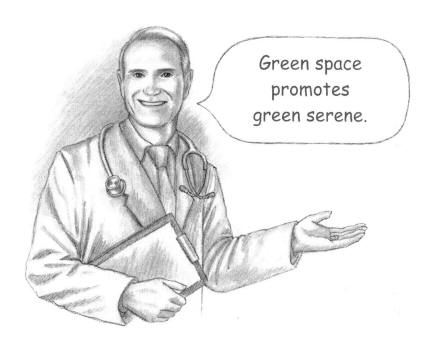

Imagine inside your body and brain you have command centers full of dials, which can be turned up or down and set just right for your physical and mental well-being. These dials are interconnected by chemical emails, hormones that enable each system to talk to the other. When you walk briskly outside, the eye-brain dial says to the heart dial: "Relax heart, you don't need to beat so hard and fast." Then it says to the intestinal dials, "Gut, feel good!" And even the pain of "-itis" illnesses lessens after a walk or swim.

To enjoy the healing effects of nature, turn your desk toward the window, put plants and an indoor fountain in your office, and frequently turn your swivel chair away from the computer screen to enjoy the window view. To avoid the humped-back posture that is overtaking the iBrains and iBacks (inflammation, anyone?) of habitual texters and smartphone gazers, here is Dr. Bill's simple back-friendly remedy: As often as possible, look out and up and say "Hi to the sky." (See more, page 212.)

EYE FEEL GREAT!

There is a scientific basis to "eye candy." Neuroscientists dub the beauties of nature "visual valium." The insightful statement, "It's pleasing to the eyes" also applies to the brain since the eye is simply an extension of the brain. A reminder I often say during my nature walks is: "Retina of the eye, feel good." Called the *retinal-hypothalamic pathway*, neurospeak for the nerves that connect the eye to the pleasure centers of the brain, this is how sunlight heals. This is why Japanese research reveals that patients whose hospital beds face the window heal faster. To enjoy this *sunlight solution* to your inflammation:

- Face your desk toward a window.

- Do your workouts facing a window.

- To keep from getting bored when sitting at a meeting in a boardroom, face a window, when possible.

When possible, add the *garden effect*. Gaze through the window at a garden.

2. If You're Going to Worry, Worry While You *Walk*.

Do You Have an iBrain or iBod? While discussing illnesses with my more techie "-itis" patients, I often help them remember inflammation as the root cause of their hurts by saying: "Joey, you have iBrain," or "Lori, you have an iBod." Naturally, they don't want to fit either of these labels, so they are motivated to do The Inflammation Solution. When we sophisticated humans moved more indoors, glued our eyes to screens and our bodies to chairs, we got more inflamed. This not-so-surprising discovery is leading more neurologists, cardiologists, rheumatologists (all the –ologists for that matter) to prescribe the timeless anti-inflammatory: go outside and play. The theologists add: go outside and *pray*. *Meditation* is the most time-tested tool for healing a hurting mind – and body.

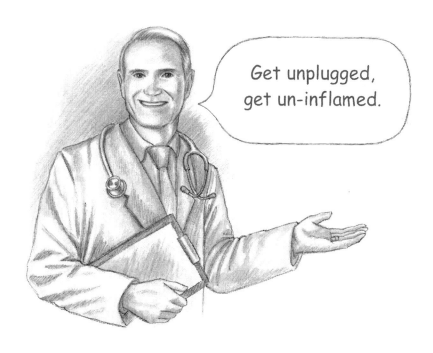

Get unplugged, get un-inflamed.

3. Swim Your Inflammation Away

Swimming is not only good for your joints (see page 211), it mellows the mind. Called "floatation therapy," swimming, or just floating, especially in warm water, seems to turn down the SNS (the "worry and run" system) and turn up the PNS (the "relax and cool it" system), helping the body regain stress balance and, therefore, inflammation balance.

4. Sleep Your Inflammation Away

Imagine sleep like taking your body and brain into a spa retreat to prevent and repair inflammation. Good sleepers tend to have better inflammation balance. During sleep your body dials down wear and tear neurochemicals: stress hormones, oxidative stress, and other sticky-stuff generators. While you rest, you heal. Mother's wisdom of "go outside and play" and "sleep well" are partners in health. Sleep

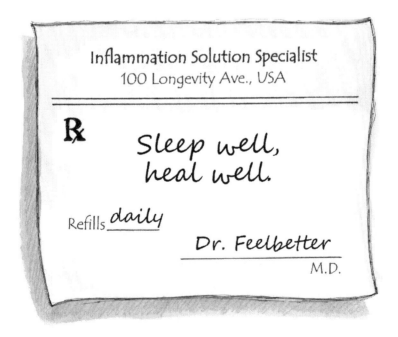

scientists believe that the reason we tend to sleep better after a day full of outdoor exercise is that during sleep, the mind replays the pleasant scenes of the day and is relaxed by what it replays. Sleep researchers theorize that the more natural sunlight your brain sees during the day, the more melatonin your brain makes at night. Quality sleep is extremely therapeutic. During slow-wave sleep, brain toxins are removed more quickly. Those who have sleep apnea or other maladies that interfere with quality of sleep often have brains that tend to age more quickly. According to Dr. Vincent Fortanasce, author of *The Anti-Alzheimer's Prescription,* if you are 40, fat, and snore, these are clues that you probably have obstructive sleep apnea (OSA) and should consult your doctor. Sleep specialists preach: "Lights down at least an hour before lights out." Bright light has an alerting effect by revving up the alertness centers of the brain, just the opposite of how you want your brain to be reset before going to bed. Avoid bright screens (computers, phones, ipads) at least an hour before bed. Turn down the bright bathroom lights. People often have bright bathroom lights to better examine their wrinkles in front of the mirror, not realizing that bright bathrooms at night can lead to poor quality sleep, which can lead to more wrinkles.

5. Breathe Your Inflammation Away

Add "take a deep breath" to mom's anti-inflammatory advice to "go outside and play." Deep breathing turns up the calming and inflammation-easing brain center, the PNS, and turns down the hyper-inflammatory response of the SNS. (For more about the feel-good effects of deep breathing, see page 226.)

6. Think Your Inflammation Away

Get rid of the "ants." "Ants," a psycho-term for *a*utomatic *n*egative *t*houghts, is the basis for the medical discovery that optimists are less inflamed than pessimists. When a negative thought enters your mind, especially a worry over which you have no control, it triggers a cascade of neurochemical pro-inflammatories that amp up your stress hormones and upset your inflammation balance. One of the hardest tools of The Inflammation Solution to use, and the one that took me the longest to master, is to get rid of negative thoughts quickly before they infect the rest of your body's inflammation balance. Here's Dr. Bill's "ant repellant": I treat negative thoughts like a negative email. I quickly send the "ants" to the imaginary "trash bin" in my brain where, hopefully, they're gone forever. I follow this with a mood-switching technique of quickly switching the mind to happy thoughts, such as a happy moment of your life (wedding day, walking on your favorite beach, your favorite dance, and so on). I use this, what I call "instant replay," to pull out of my happy-thought toolbox competing thoughts that overshadow the disturbing ones.

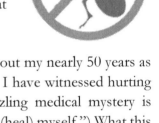

Convince yourself you will heal. Throughout my nearly 50 years as a physician, along with many other doctors, I have witnessed hurting patients willing themselves well. This puzzling medical mystery is called the *placebo effect* (Latin for "I will please (heal) myself.") What this effect really means is, "When I think I will feel better, I will feel better."

So real and so strong is the placebo effect that once upon a time, many pills to heal ills exerted much of their healing effect because the pill takers imagined, "When I take this pill, I will feel better," and they did. Because the placebo effect is so powerful, the FDA now requires drugs to be tested against a placebo, or "sugar pill," a look-alike, taste-alike pill. Only after proving the real pill outperforms the placebo pill, and the healing effects outweigh the harmful effects, is the drug approved. Because of this more objective testing requirement, many new drugs fail the test and are not approved. Mood and behavior-changing medications are particularly vulnerable to the placebo effect.

The desire, and often the desperation, to feel better cause the mind to beg the body to will the pill to work.

A fascinating new field of mind medicine is called *psychoneuroimmunology*. That mouthful means: The mind sends a neurochemical email to the brain, "I'm going to feel better." The brain listens and sends out its own chemical messengers, hormones, to the immune system, which responds by sending out its own inflammation-balancing biochemicals. Yes, you have a lot of body talk going on inside.

The placebo effect and the placebo person. Not only does popping a pill exert a powerful placebo effect, so does the prescriber. When a doctor or therapist prompts the patient, "Take this (or do this) and you'll feel better…" the patient usually does. The opposite and negative mind-over-inflammation effect is called the *nocebo* effect, or "It won't work and I won't get better." And, sadly, this downer often becomes a self-fulfilling prophecy.

Science shows the placebo effect is real. Recent studies shed some light on this medical mystery of how the mind heals the body by stimulating the brain to release natural pain relievers. To test whether the placebo effect is due to the release of feel-good hormones, such as endorphins, researchers gave subjects a drug that blocks endorphin receptors (the parking spots on the cell membranes that enable endorphin molecules to park there and relieve the pain). The placebo effect was blunted. Ah ha! More proof that the mind can prompt the body and brain to make its own medicines – the top theme of this book.

New neuroimaging technology is further proving that the mind can will the brain and body to feel better, proving there really is a neurochemical basis for "willpower." Using positron emission tomography (PET) scans – a nuclear medicine camera, like a window into the brain activity to reveal what's going on in there – research showed that when persons were injected with a saltwater placebo that they believed was a pain-killing drug, the regions of their brain involved in making and releasing the body's own natural pain-killers lighted up on the scans. Wow!

The placebo effect is not *just* "imagining" and "all in your mind." Real physical effects happen. Simply put, the mind can open or close the pharmacy within your brain and body. As a doctor, I believe the placebo effect is so powerful because the person taking the placebo feels *in control*. When the mind believes it's in control of the body, the body responds by feeling better.

The "*m*ake *y*our *o*wn *m*edicines" (MYOM) effect is particularly healthful in emotional mood disorders and neurodegenerative diseases, such as Parkinson's, which are now considered part of the ever-widening spectrum of inflammatory diseases.

Research reveals that Parkinson's, an increasingly prevalent neurodegenerative disease, is due to a deficiency in the nerve-modulating neurochemical dopamine. When neuroscientists gave persons with Parkinson's a saltwater placebo (they thought they were getting a dopamine-stimulating drug), the dopamine-producing area in the brain (the basal ganglia, the area that balances fine motor activity) actually lighted up as if increasing natural dopamine secretion, and their characteristic quirky muscle movements lessened.

Even better news, the placebo effect (natural medicines released) is greatest in those medical conditions in which pharmacologic medications show the most harmful side effects, such as in neurodegenerative diseases, mood disorders, and osteoarthritis. These discoveries are leading many neuroscientists to conclude that the "feel better" effect of many mood-altering medications is mostly due to the person's own placebo effect more than the pharmacologic effect of the prescription drug.

The real placebo effect presents real challenges to doctors prescribing medications. The doctor wants the patient to feel better and the patient desperately wants to feel better. They often could not care less whether it's due to the doctor's drug or the patient's mind.

BE HAPPY, DON'T HURT!

Carrying on the central theme of this book, help your body make its own medicines, happy feelings produce more *serotonin*. This mood-mellowing neurochemical acts like a pain-perceiving thermostat. When you turn serotonin up, you turn down pain perception.

The nocebo effect – "I will feel worse" – is as real as the "feel better" placebo, and explains a doctor's natural reluctance to tell the patient the pill may cause uncomfortable side effects, such as nausea, headache, muscle pains, and more. The mind is likely to prompt the brain and body to actually feel the discomforts. Perhaps that's why drug companies in their clever TV ads present the good news about the drug so happily and the bad news in such rapid-fire, subdued language that the viewer and listener is more positively than negatively affected by the ad.

CHAPTER 7

Self-Help for the ABCDs: Arthritis, Bronchitis, Colitis, Cognitivitis, and Dermatitis

Since the majority of "-itis" illnesses fall into these five categories, we're going to take you through a self-help plan to heal your hurts. Besides the health habits that are specific for each of these "-itis" illnesses, there are five habits that help prevent and heal all "-itis" illnesses.

JOINT HEALTH REVIEW

Here's a summary of the anti-inflammatory prescription you learned in the earlier chapters. Review it and do it:

1. Follow the six-S anti-inflammatory diet, at least six days a week (page 39).
2. Graze / enjoy the rule of twos (page 117).
3. Stay lean (page 163).
4. Do joint-friendly exercises at least an hour a day (page 199 – 221).
5. Enjoy stress control (page 180).

ALLEVIATE YOUR ARTHRITIS

Fifty-two (52) million Americans now suffer from some form of arthritis. Wow! That's a lot of hurts. Arthritis is the number one cause of chronic pain and affects over 30 percent of adults. Another shocking statistic is that Americans spend more on anti-inflammatory pain-killers than any other country. And it's ironic that the most popular drugs, such as the NSAIDs, also have the most unpopular side effects. (See The Problem with Pills," page 12.)

Besides being the most common and debilitating "-itis" illness, arthritis of the joints is easier to prevent than treat. Once severe inflammation occurs in the joint so that the surface of the joint wears away and you have bone rubbing against bone, it is very unlikely to self-repair, unlike other tissues such as skin and muscle. Severely inflamed joints often need to be replaced because they can't be repaired.

Another reason joint health is so crucial for health and longevity is that joint-itis often leads to a downward spiral: sore joints, hurts to move, sit more, get more inflamed, get bigger belly, hurts more to move, sit even more, get even more inflamed.

Next, you will notice that most inflammation occurs at the entry points where germs and toxins get into, or collect in, the body: the lining of the lungs, the intestines, the joints, and the skin. Fortunately, that's where most of the inflammatory soldiers are stationed, like checkpoints for foreign toxins that try to get in. Naturally, most of the fights ("-itis" illnesses) occur in these areas. The good news is that the organs most likely to get inflamed are also the ones most equipped with the natural ability to make their own medicines.

THINK PREVENTION

Unlike your muscles, skin, and other highly vascular tissues that easily repair themselves, joints do not, mainly because joints do not have a rich vascular network to deliver healing nutrients. They depend upon seepage of nutrients from surrounding tissues. Of all the organs of the body, prevention of joint inflammation is one of the most important because joints are the slowest to repair. This is why your friendly neighborhood orthopedist is in the joint-replacement business.

What You Need To Know About Your Knees

What's good for the knees is good for all your joints. I chose to go into detail about the knee joint because it is one of the most disabling joint problems from arthritis. Each year in the United States, 200,000 to 250,000 people undergo knee replacements. It is one of the most important joints affected by inflammation because a person disabled by arthritis of the knees moves less and sits more, which leads to more inflammation and more "-itises" throughout the body. Also, it is the most fascinating joint for appreciating the beautiful biomechanics of how your body is made.

Mobility without pain is what we all want. The average person flexes their knee joint five to ten thousand times a day. When two areas constantly rub against one another that much, wear and tear may occur. When inflammation attacks the joint surfaces, it accelerates the sticky stuff that accumulates there, worsening the already rough surface and making it even more stiff and sticky. The two structures most involved in a healthy knee joint are the *articular cartilage*, meaning the cushion that covers the bones, and the synovial membrane, the smooth and slippery-as-ice surface that covers these cushions. The more cushiony the cushions and the more slippery the surface, the more comfortably your joint moves. The more stiff and sticky it gets, the more it hurts and the less it moves. Let's examine these two fascinating structures. By appreciating how wonderfully they are designed, hopefully you'll be more motivated to take better care of them. Since inflammation of the bone, called osteoarthritis, most affects the cartilage, let's start there.

How your joint cushions work. Articular cartilage is so called because in orthopedics lingo, when joints move against each other they are said to "articulate." Articular cartilage is like a quarter-inch-thick cushion attached to the ends of the bones that acts as a "shock absorber" when you jump, dance, run, and walk. Orthopedists refer to articular cartilage as an "elastic sponge." Composed mostly of water, this firm sponge is soaked by a lubricating and anti-inflammatory fluid that has the consistency of an egg white, called synovial fluid that your joints continually squirt out. When you take a step, the weight of your body on your knees squeezes the fluid out of the sponge, which helps distribute and lessen the load pressure on your joints. When the pressure on the joint is relieved, such as between steps, the sponge naturally expands and soaks up more water to get it ready for cushioning the next step.

How your joint cushions heal. The articular cartilage, or sponge, doesn't have any blood vessels of its own, so it relies on the vascular system of the bone beneath it to continually squirt growth and repair nutrients into it. The fascinating part of the articular cartilage is how it functions as a cushion. Putting pressure on the vascular system of the bone beneath the articular cartilage compresses and releases the vascular area of the bone, allowing the articular cartilage to suck up nutrients from the underlying bone. The magnificently made knee joint is one of the few joints that the more you move it, the better it works, and the longer it lasts.

Collagen proteins, specifically chondroitin and proteoglycans, have unique qualities that make them spongy enough to act like your knee's shock absorbers, yet are firm and elastic enough to hold the cartilage tissue together. Picture strands of proteins, like magnets, on top of one another. As these magnet-like proteins get close to one another, such as happens when the cartilage sponge is compressed while taking a step, they repel one another, and the repelling force acts as a joint cushion. This also lessens the pressure on the underlying bone, which is itself rich in blood vessels and acts as a shock absorber. If it weren't for the articular cartilage, we wouldn't be able to walk for 80 or 90 years — our joints wouldn't last that long.

In a healthy joint, the articular cartilage continually repairs itself as it wears out. When some magnets wear out, other new magnets appear. Yet, as we age, two problems occur in the sponge. The first is that the cartilage cells, called chondrocytes, lessen their ability to make new and younger cells when the old ones wear out. The second is that the sponge loses chondroitin, making it stiffer and less able to suck up synovial fluid to keep it spongy. Basically, your joint shock absorbers wear out. Also, your natural joint lubricant, synovial fluid, gets stickier, like motor oil left unchanged.

Another way to think of the cushions that surround your joint is like a balloon that continually inflates and compresses with weight-bearing and release. You take a step and you compress the balloon; between steps, the balloon re-expands. Over time, the balloon gets stiffer, and does not contract and expand as much, causing more wear and tear and less cushioning of the underlying joint. To fully appreciate how your joints work, imagine your joint cushions like walking on a waterbed. The bed compresses and relaxes with each step.

Why your joint cushions like movement. Here are two reasons why joints are meant to move. Cartilage itself does not contain blood vessels, so it depends on nourishment from the underlying, highly vascularized bone tissue upon which it sits. When you move your joints, such as flexing your knee, this movement draws growth and repair nutrients from the underlying bone into the articular cartilage cushion and other joint supporting structures by osmosis. When you don't move your joints, you essentially starve them of nutrients, causing them to get stiff, less cushiony, and eventually painful. Both ends of your knee bones (the upper bone called the femur and the lower bone called the tibia or shin bone) are covered by articular cartilage cushions.

To appreciate articular cartilage, next time you're eating a chicken or turkey dinner – and after you enjoy eating the meat off the leg bone – look at the white shiny coating of cartilage on the joint surface of the leg bone. Feel how smooth it is even after being cooked. Pull the drumstick off the thigh bone and notice the white, shiny, smooth surface on top of the drumstick where it fits into the thigh bone. Orthopedists often use this analogy to describe arthritis of the joint: take a knife and scrape the shiny articular surface of the drumstick and feel the roughness you've created. Imagine that rough surface moving 10,000 times a day. Gradually you're going to wear off the protective cartilage, leaving rough bone to slide against rough bone – ouch! In fact, this cartilage is how chicken soup gets its deserved reputation for healing. Presumably, when you cook cartilage and bones you eat nutrients that help repair your own bones. Sorry, but canned chicken soup doesn't count. It has to have the broth from the real bones.

The magnificent medicine your moving joints make. Let's take a look inside one of the most active joints in your body, the knee joint, and learn what happens when you walk.

In Chapter Four, you learned that your body is a giant walking pharmacy. While the main pharmacy resides in the blood vessels, (see page 156) you have mini pharmacies inside your joints. Like plastic wrap around your joints, a thin tissue, called the synovial membrane, encapsulates your main joints, especially hardworking joints like the knee. The medicine this membrane makes is called *synovial fluid*. Picture your joint being continually bathed in a protective, anti-inflammatory fluid.

Synovial fluid helps joint health in three ways:

- It *lubricates*. Synovial fluid provides a slippery surface to lessen wear and tear of bones sliding over each other as happens in the knee joint five to ten thousand times a day in the average walker.

- It *nourishes*. Sort of like blood does to muscle, it delivers nutrients and removes metabolic waste.

- It acts like a *shock absorber*. What makes this fluid so fascinating is that it changes viscosity when it needs to protect the joint surfaces. When you stand, walk, or apply any weight to the joint, this shock-absorbing fluid automatically becomes thicker to absorb some of the weight off the bone surfaces. Then when you sit and rest the joints, this fluid also "rests" by becoming thinner. Wow, what a design!

The lining of the synovial membrane continuously secretes and absorbs fluid, keeping it fresh. This magical membrane sucks the fluid and nutrients it needs from the tiny blood vessels supplying the joint, and then squirts fresh fluid into the joint. It also sucks the waste back out of the joint fluid into the blood vessels.

Next time you take a step, imagine your knee joint saying, "I'm making my own medicines." Synovial fluid makes your joints spongier. If it weren't for synovial fluid and the spongy, slippery design of the bone surfaces of the joint, we'd all be stiff, sore, and arthritic, even in childhood.

How movement makes joint medicine. One of the central inflammation-balancing themes of this book is that the body is made to move, especially for joint health. Here's what happens when you do one of my favorite joint-healing exercises – knee pumping – and even during simple walking. Flexing and extending your knees, like during walking or pumping, causes pressure changes between the fluid in the blood vessels and the fluid within the joint, increasing the movement of fluid from joints back into the blood vessels and blood vessels back into the joints, thus insuring more removal of the waste products of metabolism and inflammation and delivery of healing nutrients. Simply put, movement makes more healing fluid go into and out of the joint faster.

The magnificent meniscus. As if the designer of joints knew that we would eventually wear them out, joints, such as the knee joint, are endowed with an extra cushion, called a meniscus. They look like two soft, spongy, cartilaginous doughnuts attached to the top of the tibia bone, that cushion the weight-bearing of the leg bones pressing against each other, such as during running and jumping (see figures, page 198). Like the articular cartilage, the meniscus is a quarter-inch thick, so you have a total of a half-inch of cushioning between the knee bones. These are the best shock absorbers in your whole body. Unfortunately, it is the knee structure that is often damaged by a sports injury. This is called a torn meniscus, such as what happens when you "twist your knee."

If you twist, you may tear. With age, the meniscus weakens and is more easily torn when you twist your body. Remember, because the cushions (articular cartilage) and menisci have poor blood supply, they are very slow to heal. Arthritis, or inflammation, of the joint is basically wear and tear and rust on the surfaces – sticky stuff. While writing this book, I tore a meniscus while swing dancing with a teen. (See "Think before you move," page 209.)

How inflammation hurts the knees. Suppose you overdo your dancing, which I have done twice, causing an "-itis" of the knees. Throughout the body there are built-in sensors, or signals, between the cells of all the tissues. When you overdo your dance steps or run without a warm-up, or in any other way injure or abuse your joints, the overused or damaged tissues send out a signal that they need help to heal. In comes your inflammation army of healing biochemicals. Inflammation really is a healing reaction to injury. First comes increased blood supply, as if the healing army needs a wider highway and more roads to bring in its healers. That's the *reddening* part of inflammation. Then comes the extra blood cells carrying healing agents, and all this extra fluid causes the area to swell. When tissues swell, they hurt, and pain is the body's signal that repair is going on in there. With arthritis, joint surfaces become stiff and sticky instead of slick and slippery, thus leading to more inflammation and injury in a sticky downward spiral.

What's in Your Knees?
Happy Knee   Hurting Knee

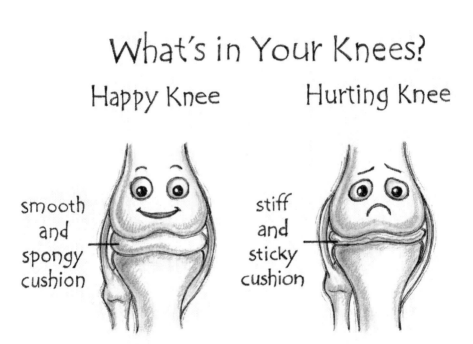

smooth and spongy cushion

stiff and sticky cushion

What's good for your knees is good for all your joints.

TEN WAYS TO BE NICE TO YOUR KNEES

1. Strengthen your supporting knee muscles. A joint is as stable as the muscles around it. The stronger the muscles supporting your knee joints, the more these muscles protect your knees from injury. Also, stronger quads and hamstrings can take some of the load off the knee joints while walking and running. (For knee-muscle strengthening exercises, see DrSearsWellnessInstitute.org/resources/inflammation /knee-exercise.)

2. Lighten the load. Stay lean. The more overweight you are, the more wear and tear on your knees. An extra pound of weight increases the pressure on your knees three-fold. Excess weight is not nice to your knees in the following ways:

- Throws your body out of balance, which causes uneven joint movement and increases wear and tear, especially on your hips and knee joints.
- Slows down your ability to move, which increases "-itises" all over your body.
- The more excess waist fat and weight you carry around, the more pressure on your arches, which causes them to "fall," leading to knock knees, which increases wear and tear on the inner joint surfaces of your knees – the most common areas for arthritis. Every pound of excess weight (fat) you lose equates to three pounds less weight pressure on your knees. That's a good return on your lean investment!

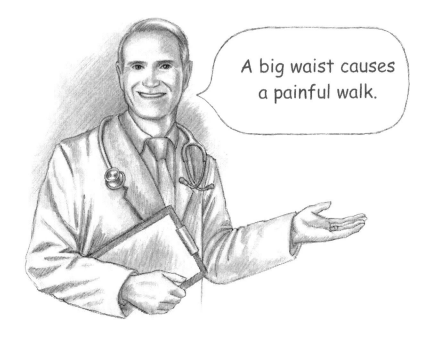

- Increases compression pressure on the knee joint with each step.
- Throws your inflammatory response out of balance. Excess belly fat spews more wear and tear chemicals into your bloodstream, and therefore into your joints. This is especially true of big waists, which causes a "waddle walk," increasing friction stress and wear and tear on the hips and knees.

3. Cushion your heels. The older you get, the softer – and lower – should be your heels. Since the foot was never designed to run on hard surfaces, I prescribe all runners, joggers, and basketball players heel cushions. Also, the older you get, the more cushioned your heels should be, especially if you are a heel pounder.

4. Walk softly. Millennia ago, our joint genes were designed to walk on sand, grass and dirt – softer surfaces – not concrete, asphalt, and hard gym floors. The knee is wired to walk, but walk with a balanced gait where your cushioned heel touches the ground slightly before the ball of your foot. Since downhill walking produces the most wear and tear and uneven pressure on your knees (the top leg bone slides in front of the lower leg bone), try avoiding downhill walking as much as possible. If necessary, walk in a *zigzag* down the hill rather than walking straight ahead. Try walking on flat surfaces as much as possible because hill walking causes a sliding motion that can be more abrasive to knee joints.

Don't pound your heels. Are you a heel pounder, walking heavily with a clomp-clomp-clomp gait? Adjust your walking to a less heel-pounding gait to ease the wear and tear on your knees. Have a friend videotape you walking or get a professional gait-analysis by a sports medicine specialist.

5. Move your joints. Joints are made to move. Arthritis 101 is the less you move, the more you hurt. Remember your joints have natural healing medicines inside called synovial fluid. Moving your joints is like squeezing the medicine bottle inside your joint and releasing healing fluid. Using the highway repair analogy, well-traveled roads need more resurfacing. Movement mobilizes the repair fluids within your knee by causing the natural sponge-like cushions to draw nourishment from the underlying bones every time they're compressed and released. My favorite movements are "knee pumping" exercises. When you move your knees, and any joint, imagine you're pumping oil that lubricates your joints. Try these knee exercises:

- Elliptical trainers
- Bicycling: stationary or moving

- Anytime / anywhere knee exercises: when standing around, hold on with one hand while pumping your knee up and down.

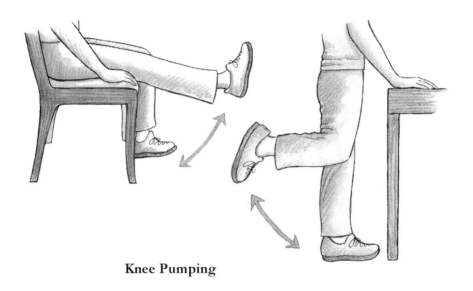

Knee Pumping

6. Swim to your knee's content. Suppose you consulted a top doc to help heal your hurting knees. You open your consultation with, "Doctor, my knees hurt so much. Please give me the safest yet most effective medicine to help my knees feel better." Top Doc reaches for her prescription pad and surprisingly scribbles out, "Swim."

Wonder why swimming works so well? Hydrotherapy is the best movement for any joint because it doesn't jar the joint; it's rhythmic, it's relaxing, and there's no pounding or twisting. Walk in water, especially if you have a leg injury. Any leg pain, such as hip, knee, or ankle, can cause you to walk off balance on land, which further aggravates the wear and tear in that joint. Walking in water takes the weight off the joint, enabling you to walk in a more balanced and normal way. Gradually progress to *marching* in water by lifting your legs higher. If painful, avoid the frog kick, which is the least friendly to sore knees. Instead, do the dolphin kick. Swimming with fins helps strengthen the tendons over the kneecaps. Call this exercise "water wellness." (See more swimming tips, page 211.)

One day I was swimming in a quiet pool and along came two friends – Dr. Vincent Fortanasce, author of *The Anti-Alzheimer's Prescription*, and his wife, Gayl, a psychotherapist. As they saw me swimming, I looked up and said, "I'm taking my anti-Alzheimer's prescription, and I'm in therapy." Actually, there is a name given to the psychological and physical benefits of swimming, *flotation therapy.*

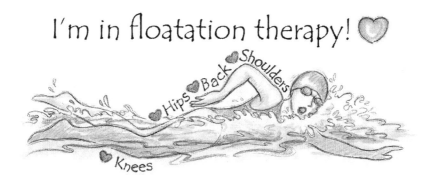

7. Nourish your knees. What you eat affects your joints. The less sticky stuff that enters your mouth, the less stiff and sticky your joints. Eat the Six-S diet as explained on page 39.

8. Wear knee-friendly shoes. The wider and more cushiony the shoe, the more stable on your knees and hips. My favorite is Grid by Saucony. For you golfers, the older you get, the shorter should be your cleats, and no cleats would be better. I wear the Saucony shoes as my golf shoes. Knee "-itises" occur when your foot is planted while your body twists. Watch a golfer with cleated shoes plant one foot while the rest of his body twists around the planted foot during the swing. As an amateur golfer I preach: The older you get, the shorter your swing and the more flexible should be your cleats. That extra few yards you will drive isn't worth the wear and tear caused by the torsion on your knees while you plant your foot. If you twist, you will shout.

9. Twist less. Again, don't do the twist in any sport! The older you get, the less you want to twist your knees and hips. For dancing, stick to waltzing instead of twisting. Both my knee injuries were due to over-twisting by trying to keep up with the younger twisters.

10. Think before you move. During the writing of this book, I gave a "Keep Your Joints Healthy" talk to teens at a dance studio. After my talk, when I had been sitting for 45 minutes, one of the dancers asked me to dance. My desire to dance was so strong that without a warm-up and without first thinking, I said, "Yes, put on *Sing, Sing, Sing*," a very knee-stressing dance. The painful inflammation of my knee finally healed two months later.

TEN TIPS FOR BUILDING BETTER BACK HEALTH

"Doctor, I've got a pain in the back!" Remember, pain is your inner voice of neurochemical emails that are released by injured or inflamed tissues, prompting you to make changes. Back pain is one of the most common reasons to visit a doctor. Spine problems are the number one reason people visit emergency rooms, the number two reason for visiting their doctor, and the third most common elective surgery in the United States. Here are some time-tested tips for preventing, or easing, pains in the back.

1. Stand smart. The older we get, the better our posture needs to be, just the opposite of the slumped over appearance of many seniors. Back Health 101 is "preserve your curve," meaning the natural S-curve in the spine, which is often compromised by poor posture when walking, standing, or sitting. Orthopedists refer to this common condition as the "postural syndrome" or "the bent back syndrome." Back pain is common in people who have a sedentary job or who habitually stand or walk slumped over. Faulty posture puts excess and uneven pressure on the disc spaces between the spinal bones, leading to weakness and inflammation of the bones and compression or rupture of the discs. And the longer you don't preserve your curve, the muscles and tissues supporting your backbones often shorten to accommodate the slumped-over posture (called adaptive shortening), causing more stress on the already inflamed back-bone joints. Try these posture-perfect changes:

- Stand straight, but not rigidly straight. The key to taking pressure off the back bone is to divert some of the weight bearing from the lower back bones to the muscles of the hips and thighs. Here's how: Stand short (slightly bend your knees instead of standing tall). By not locking your knees and instead bending them slightly, you transfer some of the weight from your back and knee joints to your thigh muscles. Remember not to lock your knees when standing.

- Use the pelvic tilt. Tuck in your buttocks and tilt your pelvis slightly forward by tightening the abdominal and buttock muscles.

- Don't arch your back while standing, as this puts excessive pressure on your backbone.

- Flex your hips while standing. Place one foot on a stool or a step while standing for long periods of time. This lessens the strain on your back.

2. Walk and stand with head up. Instead of slumping over and looking at the ground while you walk, keep your chin parallel to the ground. One of the oldest posture-perfecting tips, perhaps one your mother always said to you, is while walking or standing, imagine a string is attached to the top of your head pulling you up toward the sky. Or, stand with your back against the wall. With proper posture, the wall should touch the back of your head, your shoulder blades, and your buttocks. Since our natural tendency is to look down when we stand or walk, safely look up at the sky as much as you can while walking, and certainly while standing. This gives the neck and back bones a natural lift, in addition to strengthening your neck and back muscles. When you have to look down while walking, move only your eyes downward without bending your neck so much.

Like standing and walking, try not to slump over while sitting and keep your head in line with your back, as if you're drawing a line down the back of your head to your back to your buttocks, and that line is the same line as the back of the chair. Just like when standing, keep in mind the trick of "imagine a string is attached to the top of your head and pulling you upright."

Dr. Bill advises: *"Say hi to the sky."* Here's why. As often as possible, say while you're standing in line or walking, gaze toward the sky for ten seconds or so. Sky gazing strengthens the posture muscles of the neck and back that have been weakened and shortened by the head-down gazing that is the posture most of us assume while working and walking.

3. Sitting tips to ease a sore back. Not only do we sit too much, another "-itis" trigger is sitting unhealthfully. If your job requires hours of sitting, here's what the back doctor orders:

Cushion your back while sitting. Using a footstool and keeping your knees slightly higher than your hips puts more weight onto your feet and thigh muscles and less on your back. Also, cushion your seat. Don't plop down suddenly on a bare-seated wooden chair. If it has no cushion, ease onto it. Better is to only use cushioned chairs or use your coat as a cushion if you need to. To preserve your curve in your back while sitting, use a cushioned backrest for your lumbar spine, or roll up a towel or jacket and place it between the curve in your lower back and the back of the chair. Lumbar cushions are great for preserving your normal back curve while sitting.

Be particularly careful when sitting on a hard seat while driving on bumpy roads, such as on a bus or ATV. Your spinal column is like a bunch of blocks stacked on top of one another with natural cushions (called discs) between them. These discs are like fluid-filled doughnuts that act as shock absorbers for the spinal bones. Constant bumping of these natural cushions while driving on a bumpy road runs the risk of inflaming or rupturing them.

Enjoy a swivel chair. Besides sitting for a shorter period of time, swivel chairs are more back-friendly. You can swivel instead of twisting your back as you turn from side to side during a conversation or get up from the chair.

Use a work chair. A work chair has the following back-friendly features. Both the backrest and the seat should be adjustable, allowing you to adjust the backrest to fit the normal lumbar curvature of your spine. Adjust the seat height so that your thighs remain horizontal without pressing into the seat. Oftentimes, adjusting the seat so that the front, or your knees, is an inch lower than the back relieves excess pressure on the lower back. Adjust the backrest to softly touch the bottom of your shoulder blades and to snugly cushion your natural lumbar

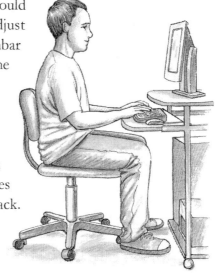

Sitting Posture - Lumbar Support

curve. Remember the golden rule of back health: preserve your curve. The more hours per day you can "preserve your curve," the better your back will feel. Prolonged sitting and bending flattens the natural lumbar curve and fatigues the supporting ligaments, setting you up for an aching back. The most common cause of back pain, and the most easily preventable, is putting the back bones in a prolonged posture, which overstretches the supporting ligaments. Overstretched tissues swell and become inflamed and hurt even more as they heal. Adjust the seat height to ease your eyes. Ideally, your eyes, when naturally gazing, are neither open too wide or closed too small. They are best rested when your line of sight matches the level of the top line of text on your monitor. Eye fatigue is greatest when you have to look up too high with eyelids wide open too long. Neck fatigue and poor posture occurs when your head is bent low to read the screen. Head erect, eyes slightly downward is the ideal neck posture.

Get up and stretch. Take periodic standing and walking breaks to take pressure off your lumbar discs, the natural cushions between your backbones.

Walk while you talk. If possible at your workplace, if you plan to be on a long phone call, talk while you walk. Plan the call at a time when you can be walking around a hallway, outdoors, or just around your private office.

4. Lift with your knees and thighs and not with your back. Besides standing, walking, and sitting smart, lift smart. Lift with your leg and hip muscles and not your back muscles. Bend your knees, but keep your back as straight as possible while lifting. Keep the heavy object as close to your body as possible during lifting so you don't have to bend your back. The same with stooping. Squat instead of stooping over. Again, keep your back straight and your knees bent.

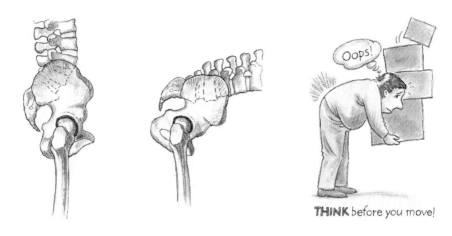

Hinge hips, don't bend back.

Always bend your knees first and not your back. Unlike other joints, the spine was not made to bend that much.

5. Carry smart. Remember, your goal is to put the weight on your leg muscles and not your back. By carrying heavy objects as close as possible to your chest and abdomen, you help your abdominal and thigh muscles bear most of the weight. Distribute the weight evenly on both sides, such as not carrying a heavy grocery bag dangling from one arm. Better to carry one lighter bag in each arm. Also, the older and more sensitive your back, the less you should use a backpack; but if you do, keep it to no more than ten percent of your body weight.

6. Lower your heels. The higher your heels, the more strain on your back. High heels encourage swayback posture that disturbs the normal S-curve of the spine.

7. Think before you move. Suddenly twisting, such as getting out of a car or hopping out of bed, torques the back bones, setting up an inflammatory response. Be particularly careful upon arising in the morning. During sleep your cushiony lumbar discs swell, making them more injury prone from sudden twisting. To get out of bed in the most back-friendly way, roll over on your side. Then, using your hands, push up your upper body to a sitting position on the side of your bed while placing your feet on the floor.

8. Sleep in a back-friendly position. Even during sleep, try to preserve your curve. Sleeping flat flattens out the curve and stresses the lower spine. Sleeping on your side is often the most back-friendly. Try putting pillows under your head, between your knees, and a small folded towel between the mattress and your waist. With back-sleeping, to preserve the curve, besides the usual neck pillow, place a large pillow under your knees and a small pillow or folded towel in the curvature of your back.

9. Stay lean. "Doctor, I've got a bad back!" "That's because you've got a big belly." One of the most stressful and "-itis"-producing postures on the natural curvature of the spine is the pelvis tilting downward caused by the big belly. When the belly hangs over the belt,

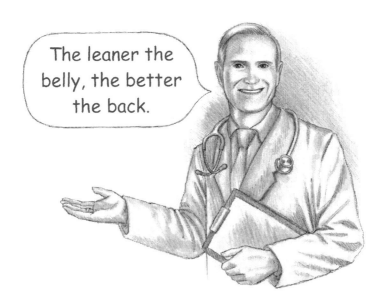

the back bone cries, "Ouch!" A big belly increases the wear and tear and arthritis on the back, hip, and knee joints.

10. Stretch and strengthen your supporting muscles. The more you strengthen your back and abdominal muscles (called core muscles), the better your back. Like all joints, the spinal bones are only as strong as the muscles supporting them. Another painful consequence of the sitting disease is what orthopedists call *adaptive shortening*. When you don't stretch and move your muscles enough, the ligaments and muscles supporting the backbones shorten and weaken. Then, when you suddenly try to stretch these tissues, they hurt.

(For safe and comfortable back-building exercises, see DrSearsWellnessInstitute.org/resources/inflammation/exercises).

SWIM TO YOUR BACK'S CONTENT

A fun and effective way to keep the hump out of your back is to swim the breast stroke. The muscle and bone position of the back and neck while swimming the breast stroke de-humps the muscles, tendons, and back and neck bones that are bent over while slumping. And, as an extra perk, looking up at the surroundings and beautiful sky while swimming helps you enjoy it more. Remember, if you have knee pain, instead of the frog-kick, which is hard on the knees, use the usual knee-pumping flex kick with the breast stroke. For another kick to strengthen back, glute, and hip muscles, scissor your straight legs from center to side and back.

BETTER-BACK EXERCISES

If you're an exercise addict, like this author, you will hear goodies like "strengthen your core" and "stabilize your trunk." This important bit of gym-rat wisdom simply means the stronger the muscles in your middle, the stronger the bones in your back. Or, putting it another way, strong belly muscles lead to strong back muscles. This correlation is because of the orthopedic truism: *Your bones and joints are only as strong as the muscles supporting them.*

AN ANYTIME / ANYWHERE EXERCISE FOR BACK HEALTH

Before we get into specific back-strengthening exercises, remember the most easily doable, anytime / anywhere posture-preserving exercise: Say hi to the sky (see below). Since most of us spend most of our days looking downward, remind yourself to look up toward the sky at least once an hour while holding your arms up or out, and hold for 10-20 seconds. You can do that!

iPosture-itis. Many of us spend hours a day humped over, peering at our smartphone or tablet, eventually leading to neck and upper back pain and inflammation. At least every 10 minutes, unbend and say "hi to the sky."

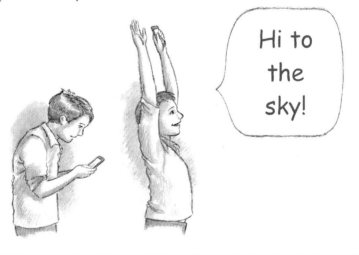

Basic core-strengthening positions while lying on your back.
Contract your abdominal muscles while pushing the lumbar curve toward the floor and hold for 10-20 seconds. While in this position, slowly bicycle your legs while maintaining the flexing and crunching of your abdominal and lumbar muscles toward the floor.

Make a bridge. While keeping the same lying-down posture, plant your feet on the floor, press heels to floor, and lift hips toward ceiling. Lift as high as you can *without arching your back*. Contract your glutes (buttock muscles) and hold for 10-20 seconds. Repeat several times. Next, while keeping your hips up, carefully extend and hold up one leg at a time, while keeping the other foot pressed to the floor.

Prone position exercises. While lying on the floor, roll over to the prone position. Put weight on your hands and knees. Suck in your abdominal muscles toward your back while lifting your hips off the floor, holding your weight on elbows and toes. Again, don't arch your lower back. Hold 10-20 seconds, and repeat ten times.

While still prone, place a pillow under your hips. Lift and hold one leg at a time while keeping knees straight. Lift your leg using primarily your buttock muscles. Then lift one arm and leg at a time. As your back muscles get stronger, play "airplane" by lifting arms out to the side, keeping your abdominal muscles pressed into the pillow and your back straight. You'll naturally feel the strengthening pressure on your lower back muscles and glutes.

Hands and knees positions. Position yourself on your hands and knees while sucking in abdominal muscles toward the back and, without arching your back, hold this position for 10-20 seconds. Next, extend one arm and the opposite leg straight out from your body and hold 10-20 seconds. Repeat with opposite arm and leg.

Ball exercises (my favorite). With your feet planted securely on the floor and the back of your shoulders on the ball, flex your glutes and lower back muscles gently up and down without arching your back. Then, with your hands on your hips, raise your shoulders (keeping head straight) while flexing your abdominal muscles. Hold for 10-20 seconds.

For the really agile, try the prone-plank position. With the ball under your legs and your hands on the ground supporting you, flex abs, glutes, and lower back muscles, again without overly arching your back.

The knee cross. While lying on your back and keeping shoulders planted to floor, place right foot under left knee and stretch right knee over the left thigh. Hold 10-20 seconds. Repeat with the other side. This is a good back-muscle stretching exercise before getting out of bed in the morning.

(Note: For photos of these back exercises and more, see DrSearsWellnessInstitute.org/resources/inflammation/back-exercises).

HAVE HEALTHY HIPS

All the health habits you learned for the knees and back also apply to hip health. To reemphasize the importance of staying lean, the top contributor to sore hips is a big belly. Besides spewing sticky inflammatory chemicals into your blood and hip joints, the off-balance "belly walk" is hard on the hips. When doctors see the red flag of a "waddle walk," that is a hip-replacement waiting to happen. (See Toxic Waist, page 164.) To enjoy happy hips, swimming, like it is for all joints, is one of the best movements for hip health (except the frog kick which can be hard on the hips and knees).

BE GOOD TO YOUR GUMS

Your mouth is a hidden source of "-itis" producers. Doctors have long recognized that the health of a person's gums can affect the health of the rest of the body. Cardiologists noticed the connection between healthy gums and a healthy heart. Periodontists call it the *perio-cardio relationship*. Translation: sore gums lead to sick hearts. Chronic gingivitis seems to rev up the pro-inflammatory system, in effect keeping the fires burning in the body and increasing the severity of "-itises" all over the body. Keep sticky stuff off your teeth: caramels, cotton candy, and hard candy. Don't *chew* vitamin C (ascorbic acid) tablets, which can erode enamel. Swallowing capsules is safer. Here's Dr. Bill's time-tested gum health regimen:

1. *Swish* with warm water or green tea after eating.

2. Use a *soft* brush twice a day, especially when arising and retiring; or use a sonic toothbrush. Use *xylitol* toothpaste. Unlike sticky sucrose toothpaste sweeteners, xylitol helps prevent oral bacteria from sticking to the teeth.

3. Use a *proxy brush* (a tiny Christmas-tree-looking gum cleaner) at the gum line between each tooth; carry one in your pocket.

4. Glide *floss* between teeth to remove any remaining sticky stuff.

5. *Scrape* tongue with scraper as far back as you can without causing gagging.

6. End with 1-2 minutes of *water flossing*, especially along the gum line.

You can do this!

SAVE YOUR SHOULDERS

Your shoulder joint, because of its 360-degree rotation range and multiple planes of movement, is the most complicated joint. Because it is often the slowest "joint-itis" to heal, prevention is the key. Besides all the general joint-health habits you learned:

Warm up cold shoulder muscles. Cold, unprepared and un-stretched muscles and tendons are more prone to injury and inflammation. Before heavy shoulder work like golf, tennis, yard work, or lifting:

- *Windmill warm-up.* Wave and rotate your arms like a windmill.
- *Massage* the front of your shoulder joint just below the end of your collarbone. Massage plus a jet of warm water from a shower or jet-bath gets more blood flow into the tissues supporting the shoulder joint, called the *rotator cuff*, which is prone to "-itis" and injury.

STRETCH OUT YOUR STIFFNESS

The more we age, the more we need to move—and stretch. Our muscles not only get weaker if we don't move them, they get shorter and tighter if we don't stretch them. Another type of patient slumping into the doctor's office is one with "stiff man syndrome."

Stretch shoulder muscles. After your warm-up, gently stretch shoulder muscles and tendons with gradually increasing intensity, especially before intense activities like tennis, golf, dancing, and lifting (See stretching exercises, page 220.) The easiest shoulder stretches are:

- Clasp hands behind back and slowly lift them up three times.
- Pull against a nearby support, such as a countertop or railing.
- Raise arms above head, palms touching, and stretch side to side, up and down.
- Grab your extended arm with your opposite arm and pull across midline.

Rest shoulder joints or change sports. Take shoulder pain as your body's prompt that you are either overusing or misusing your joints, such as in a tennis, golf, bowling, or baseball swing. Take a few days rest from these sports. Swim and walk instead. The natural dangling, swing action of the arms during rhythmic walking is just what the shoulder doctor ordered.

Lift smart. Be vigilant when lifting up or taking down heavy airline carry-on baggage. The straining to get it up into the overhead compartment and bringing it down can twist and inflame back and shoulder muscles.

GET FIT WHILE YOU SIT

Are you ready to learn the easiest fitness tip that anyone can do anytime and anywhere? You don't need a gym or weights, nor is there anything to buy. You just need to hold groups of muscles flexed until you feel "the burn," usually one to two minutes. Exercise physiologists give this fitness strategy scientific names, such as: *isometrics* (muscles that flex but don't move), and NEAT (*n*on-*e*xercise *a*ctivity *t*hermogenesis – burning calories while you're sitting or standing). As a graduate from a hyperactive child to a hyperactive adult, these anytime/anywhere exercises are one of my favorite ways to keep lean and fit.

Since much of this book was written in the air, especially during a recent around-the-world-in-20-days lecture tour, including 53 hours on airplanes, here's how I kept muscles toned and burned a few indulgent calories.

Flex while you sit:

- Flex your feet up and down and pump your knees.

- Put one ankle over the other; push down with top leg and push up with the bottom leg. This isometrically flexes both the quads and the hamstrings, the muscles that support the knees.

GET FIT WHILE YOU SIT *(CONT'D)*

- Hold these isometric flex positions for 30-60 seconds or until you feel "the burn."

- Stretch your feet out underneath the seat in front of you. Push up your toes against the bottom of the seat and hold for 30-60 seconds, or until your quads feel the burn. During isometrics you'll notice your pulse and breathing increase, proving that you really are "exercising" without even leaving your seat.

- For shoulder and elbow muscle health, place one palm over the other wrist. Push down with upper arm and up with bottom arm. Reverse arms and repeat.

- Cup one fist with other hand. Push one arm against the other while also flexing your pectoral muscles.

- While standing in line for the bathroom on one of those bladder-inconsiderate planes (one lavatory to 60 passengers) stretch to your joints' content. Stand quietly on your tiptoes with your knees slightly bent and hold that position for 20-30 seconds or until you feel the burn. You'll notice that the front of your thigh muscles, the quads (the main supporting muscles of the knee joint), get a good workout.

While standing in line at the airline counter before an international flight, I stood on my flexed toes, did some slight up and down movements, as well as upper arm and pectoral-flexing isometrics. From a distance, I must have looked like a flying phobic. A nice attendant offered, "Sir, if you're afraid of flying, we have counselors that can help you." When I told her about my anytime, anywhere workout, we both laughed.

STRETCH THE BANDS

For an easy anytime/anywhere workout, a stretch band is part of my fitness prescription. Safer than free weights, they are easy on the joints while still strengthening muscles. While traveling, I carry my "anti-inflammation band" in a suitcase. While waiting for the plane and while watching sports on television, I have enjoyed many minutes of muscle-flexing.

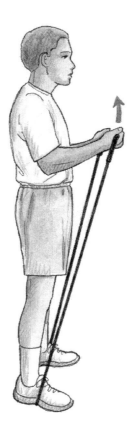

SUGGESTED STRETCHING EXERCISES

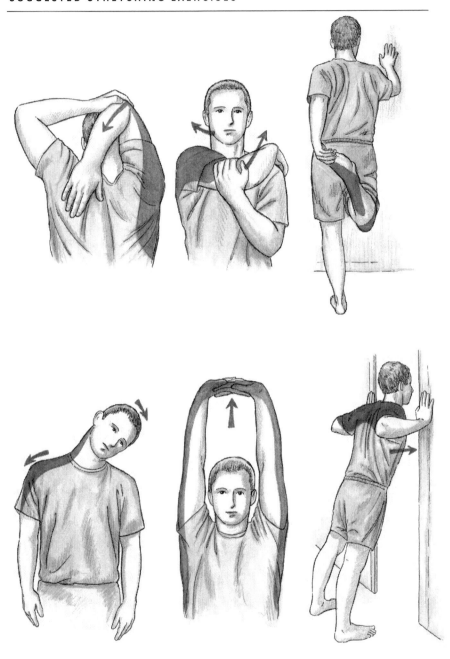

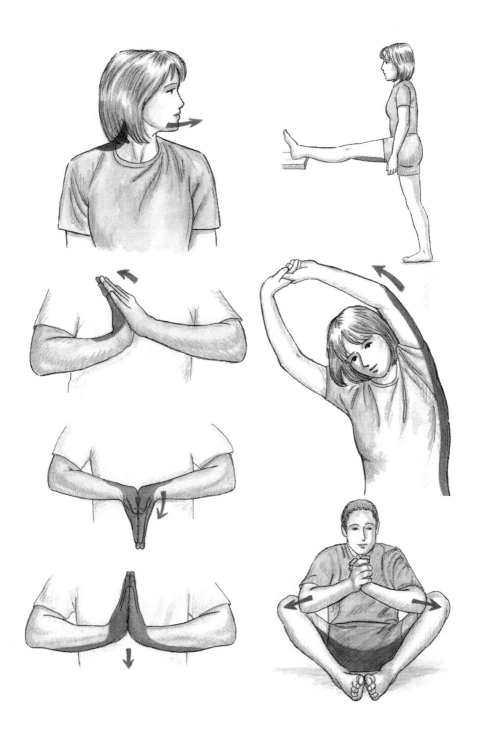

BRONCHITIS

The lining of your breathing passages are especially prone to "-itis" illness (bronchitis) because it is the first entry point of air-borne germs and toxins. Let's follow an "-itis"-causing germ or allergen to see how it gets through the airway checkpoints into the lower airways and triggers an excessive anti-inflammatory response.

First, a germ or allergen floats into the nose. If it doesn't get trapped there, it makes its way down into the bronchi. Fortunately, lining the bronchi like a shaggy carpet, are millions of tiny "police," called cilia, meaning hair. Think of cilia as miniature police waving big fans against polluted air saying, "Get out! You don't belong here!" But some intruders may get through. So, beneath the cilia is a layer of mucus that acts like protective paint to trap foreign invaders. Called *muco-ciliary clearance*, this traps invaders and, like a conveyer belt, the cilia wave the foreigners back up into the airway. The cilia act like brooms to sweep the invaders back up and out, and the mucus acts like a magnet catching dust, germs, and irritants that get past the cilia. When the dust settles, shall we say, the cilia and mucus call for help. Enter the cough reflex, which bellows the bad stuff up and out of the lungs.

If the irritants or germs get past the muco-ciliary barricade or stay there too long, the fight that breaks out (inflammation) can trigger a systemic excess inflammatory response and release pro-inflammatories that constrict the airways, making it difficult to breathe: asthmatic bronchitis.

Besides over-responding with excess inflammation that triggers wheezing, it creates too much mucus that becomes too thick. This triggers a chronic cough to keep this sticky stuff from getting stuck in the lower airways or down into the lung tissues. Remember, germy mucus, like water in a stagnant pond, gets infected (pneumonitis or pneumonia). Over time, repeated exaggerated inflammatory responses damage lung tissue, leading to chronic obstructive pulmonary disease (COPD), or stiff and sticky lung tissue.

The Anti-Inflammatory Lung Prescription

Your anti-bronchitis prescription is to keep the air you breathe clean, your nose clear, and the muco-ciliary action just right. Here's how:

1. Breathe clean air. No smoking, please. You all know that! Go out of your way to avoid travelling behind a bus spewing out exhaust fumes. When possible, think before you expose yourself to polluted air. If you have a dusty bedroom, use a HEPA air filter. You inhale around 600 breaths per hour. Over a year, that's a lot of either clean or dirty air entering your lungs.

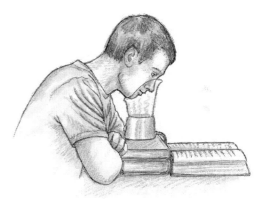

Steam clean

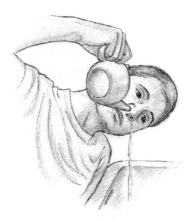

Nose hose

2. Keep your nose and sinuses clean. Your sinuses and nasal cavities both warm and slightly filter the air before it gets into the bronchi. Try Dr. Bill's home remedy: a *nose hose* and *steam clean.* A *neti pot* and *facial steamer* is just what the pulmonologist (another "-ologist" for another "-itis") ordered.

3. Humidify the air. But not too much. Central heating dries out the muco-ciliary action. In your bedroom, turn down dry central heat and turn up one or two vaporizers, which act as a heat source and moistens the air. Using a hygrometer, (available at a hardware store), try to keep the humidity around 50 percent. Much higher may produce *mold*. By the way, chronic mold collecting in damp areas of your home is one of the hidden triggers of chronic bronchitis.

LUNG CHANGES WITH AGING

Yes, it's those "old words" again: stiff and sticky. As we age, some loss of lung tissue usually occurs, but when and how much is under your control:

- **Air sacs get stiffer.** Your lungs are filled with millions of tiny balloons, called alveoli or air sacs, which inflate and deflate with each breath.

- **Blood supply gets stiffer.** The capillaries, those tiny vessels that circle the air sacs and ferry oxygen to the bloodstream, may get stiff, sticky, and less open.

- **Rib cage stiffens.** Because the muscles and bones of your chest may stiffen, you may be less able to take a deep breath.

- **Airway-lining immunity weakens.** The muco-ciliary conveyor belt may not work as efficiently to remove irritants.

Big belly restricts breathing. People with big bellies have more difficulty taking big breaths. And excess fat that accumulates around the upper airways can partially obstruct air entry while sleeping, a situation called obstructive sleep apnea.

4. Enjoy natural mucolytics. Mucolytics (mucus looseners) help keep your muco-ciliary lining healthy:

- Enjoy steam rooms with a bit of eucalyptus.
- Garlic is a natural mucolytic. Those smelly fumes from that garlic-infused pasta you ate seem to like getting into the lining of lung tissue. (See garlic, page 81.)
- *Hydration.* Drink enough fluids to keep yourself from feeling thirsty. Then drink at least one more glass.

5. Take a deep breath. Just like you stretch your muscles to keep them from getting short and stiff, deep belly-breathing expands the lung and rib-cage tissues to keep them from getting stiff, which often happens as you age.

6. Move! Like it is for all the other "-itis" illnesses, movement is good medicine for inflamed lungs. Exercise:

- Releases natural anti-inflammatories.
- Increases number and openness of alveolar capillaries.
- Increases aerobic capacity, the ability to breathe in more oxygen.
- Strengthens the heart muscle, enabling the heart to pump more blood through stiff lung tissues.

7. Stay lean. As with all the "-itis" illnesses, the leaner your body, the better you'll breathe.

Are antihistamines all right? To stop that annoying sneeze triggered by histamine, why not just pop an antihistamine pill? Once you appreciate how marvelously your body is made to protect the respiratory tract, you might not want to pop a pill so quickly. Since most of the germs and pollutants enter our body through the

DR. BILL'S DEEP-BREATHING PRESCRIPTION

At least ten times each day, especially when you hurt or are stressed:

- Breathe in deeply from the belly. First, feel your belly expand, then your chest.

- Breathe in deeply through your *nose* for a count of five. Exciting research reveals that nasal breathing triggers the lining of the nasal and sinus tissues to release NO (see page 153) which is a natural healing and anti-inflammatory biochemical. NO is one of the most important "medicines" your body makes. Besides acting as a natural anti-inflammatory, NO acts as a vasodilator to open arteries wider, which helps the blood vessels in the lungs carry more healing oxygen to the hurting tissues.

- Hold your breath for a count of five.

- Exhale slowly for a count of five; either through your nose or through pursed lips, which keeps the lungs expanded longer to deliver more healing oxygen.

Humming heals. Humming causes the air in your nasal and sinus cavities to oscillate more, which, research proves, releases more healing NO into your airways.

breathing passages, it makes sense that the immune system would be on high alert in these areas. For example, during ragweed season you're walking through a field and some pollen enters the upper airways, triggering a sneeze, or perhaps a wheeze and a cough. Here's how your natural defenses go into action.

First, the mucus glands that line the surface of the airways secrete natural protein antibiotic-like substances called *defensins*. These glands also secrete mucus, which traps the bacteria and allergens. Then millions of tiny "brooms," called cilia, sweep the mucus (or airway garbage) up and out, often triggering a sneeze, a blow, or a cough. In pulmonary lingo, this is known as *protective mucociliary action.* Picture the sinuses, the Eustachian tubes, and the lower breathing passages all sweeping their little rivers up toward the throat where we can either swallow the mucus and let the stomach and intestines dispose of it, or cough it out. Damaging – or nourishing – any one of these protective mechanisms is going to affect airway health. The "histamine response" is really a self-protective and self-cleaning mechanism. Because it's often a natural and healthy biological effect, you don't always want to think pharmacologically and interfere with it. Instead, think biologically and sometimes go along with it. It's best to consult your doctor to avoid overusing antihistamines.

COLITIS

Like the lungs, the intestines are a security checkpoint for germs, "-itis"-producing food chemicals, and other inflammatory toxins trying to enter the body. As if Dr. Mother Nature knew that humans would abuse their gut more than any other organ, most of the body's immune system (inflammation fighters) resides in the lining and walls of the intestines. Yet, the gut is also the major checkpoint where inflammatory fights breakout. Could there be a correlation between the epidemic of chemical foods (fake foods) and intestinal "-itises"? Doctors think so.

As you learned in Chapter One, the body's intestinal police are always on the lookout for imposters (fake food). These intestinal inflammatory police are working overtime saying: "The stuff in these foods *isn't real.* Let's kick them out." Over time, because there is too much fighting going on down there, eventually there is too much wear and tear and battle fatigue, and you get an "-itis" or a "-tion":

- Indiges*tion*: heartburn

- Constipa*tion*
- Malabsorp*tion*
- Irrita*tion*: irritable bowel syndrome
- Rejec*tion*: celiac, gluten intolerance
- Inflamma*tion*: colitis, ileitis

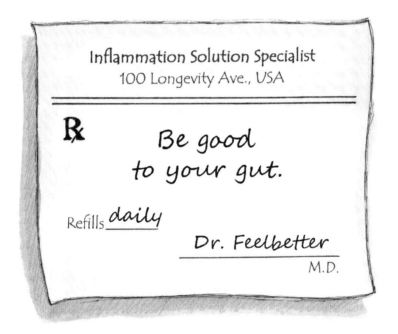

Is your gut leaking? The epidemic of "leaky gut" disease is thought to be due to fake food poking holes in the sensitive intestinal lining. This allows germs and foreign chemicals to seep through into the tissues and trigger inflammation. Inflammation and aging are the two main triggers of a leaky gut. Normally, the gut is a fine filter, allowing only healthful food molecules, and those with the right chemical makeup, to seep through the tight junctions between the cells lining the intestines. Inflammation widens the spaces between these cells, allowing larger food molecules and toxins to leak through. The nearby immune system, like roadside police, conclude, "You don't belong here, we're going to kick you out!" Hence, inflammatory bowel disease.

As a review of what you have already learned, here's the Inflammation Solution for these "shuns:"

1. Eat real food: (See why, page 35.) One of our Health Coaches (Thanks, Kathy Bee!) summed up the good gut feelings from eating real food:

   - Eat real food.
   - Poop real often.
   - Feel real good.

   You can do that!

2. Graze, the rule of twos (see page 117).

3. Enjoy the sipping solution (see page 57).

4. Eat more seafood, less animal foods (see page 46).

5. Enjoy the six-S anti-inflammatory diet (see page 39).

6. Replace fork with chopsticks (see page 118).

7. Eat less. Go for quality over quantity (see page 124).

8. Stop eating when you're 80 percent full. I learned this gut-friendly way of eating while lecturing in Okinawa (Okinawans have longer lifespans and suffer from fewer "-itis" illnesses than anyone else in most of the world). There is around a 20-minute delay for the stomach to tell the brain, "Enough already, you're full, stop eating!" When you stop short of "feeling full" and give your brain time to catch-up to the stomach, you'll eat less and yet feel satisfied.

9. Don't chargrill or overcook your food (see page 132).

10. Move your body to move your bowels.

11. Relax your gut brain (see page 125).

ARE LEAKY GUT AND LEAKY BRAIN PARTNERS IN INFLAMMATION?

Why do so many persons of all ages, from autism to Alzheimer's, have "-itis" illnesses in both brain and belly? New insights reveal the same cause – inflammation. Because of the recent findings that many children with autism also suffer from a "leaky gut," Autism Spectrum Disorder (ASD) is now considered in the spectrum of an autoimmune disease.

COGNITIVITIS

Neuroinflammation (see page 174) is overtaking aging Americans, and there are not enough neurologists to care for them. Because there are fewer pain fibers within brain tissue, slowly smoldering inflammation of the brain can build up before you realize it. This is unlike a pain in the gut or joint, which are often early clues to illness. Why are bad things happening to good brains? Here's why: the smartest organ is the one most vulnerable to inflammation.

We are "fatheads." The brain is 60 percent fat and fat tissue is the most vulnerable to inflammation if it is not protected. Have you ever mistakenly left a raw fatty fish out overnight? It oxidizes, turns rancid, or whatever you want to call it – it stinks!

Brains rust. The brain, a symphony of 100 billion neurons, is one of the most metabolically active organs in the body. It uses around 20-25 percent of all the food energy we consume and the oxygen we breathe.

The more food energy and oxygen-burning an organ needs (oxidation), the more inflammation it produces. Remember, excess oxidation is rust. Like unpainted metals exposed to air rust, unprotected brains rust.

Brains leak. Because brain tissue is so vulnerable to attack, it is protected by a one-cell-thick layer called the *blood-brain barrier*, perfectly placed between the blood vessels and brain tissue to prevent inflammatory toxins and chemicals from getting through. The BBB weakens over time, becoming a leaky barrier.

Normally *neurotoxins* that squirm through the leaky BBB are blocked from entering the inside of the brain cell by the protective cell membrane. But over time, the brain cell membrane, which is mostly fat, can weaken, resulting in a condition called *leaky cell membrane.*

Brain produces less anti-rust protection. To add more neurodegeneration to the inflaming brain, as we age the body produces more attacking inflammatory chemicals and less protective ones. The hippocampus, the area of attention and concentration, emotional content and memory is the area most attacked by Alzheimer's disease. The hippocampus is the most vulnerable area of the brain because it has the most highly metabolizing cells, needing the most blood supply and energy. Because it is the most vulnerable it needs the most antioxidant protection.

Brains get stressed out. Nervous tissue does not cope well with excess stress hormones that remain too high for too long, a degenerating effect called *glucocorticoid neurotoxicity.* Sounds like something you don't want to get. It's those darn dials again. Normally, when stress hormones get too high for too long, the brain automatically dials them down. This dial-down protective mechanism lessens with age. Yes, there are smart ways to prevent, delay, or stop progression of this debilitating disease.

Brains shrink. If we don't use and feed them right, studies reveal that sticky inflammatory biochemicals like HbA1c (see page 21) can shrink brain size.

Grain brain. Go off gluten? We've heard of wheat belly. Gastroenterologists have long known about gluten sensitivity causing a pain in the gut. While gluten, Latin for *"glue"* (i.e., sticky stuff), is being implicated in a wide variety of intestinal illnesses, Neurologists are now suspecting that gluten may also be to blame for giving you sticky stuff in the brain.

Prominent neurologist Dr. David Perlmutter, author of the must-read book *Grain Brain*, makes a science-supported case that gluten-sensitivity could be a cause of inflammation in the brain. Inflammation researchers came to this conclusion using the emerging science of nutragenetics, how food affects our genes. Our ancestors, and our genes, grew up eating a diet high in healthy fats, moderate in protein, and relatively low in carbs – or at least factory-made carbs. Around 10,000 years ago, we began eating an increasing amount of wheat. It was relatively plentiful and cheap. Yet the food-gene specialists speculate that since our genes were not originally programmed to welcome wheat into our bodies, it may take many centuries for some genes to change their mind about welcoming wheat. The modern genes of many people still regard wheat as a foreign food and, therefore, fight against it, causing inflammation.

Science supports this wheat-gene confusion:

- People with high blood sugar, usually from eating too much processed grains, have more diabetes and brain inflammation.
- The same pro-inflammatory sticky chemicals that go up in gluten-sensitive persons also may increase sticky stuff (aka "tangles," "amyloid") in persons with neurodegenerative diseases.

- Eating excess wheat is one of the top causes of high blood sugar, and the longer your blood sugar stays high, the greater your risk of Alzheimer's.

- High carbs, especially those in fake foods, not healthy fats, are more likely to contribute to Alzheimer's.

- People with higher cholesterol are *less* likely to suffer neurodegenerative diseases.

- There is a growing concern among neurologists about the possible degenerating effects of cholesterol-lowering drugs on brain function.

At this writing, like most of my family, I am eating less gluten in favor of quinoa, brown rice, amaranth, buckwheat, millet and oats. (Note: if you are severely gluten intolerant, you will want to only eat oats certified as gluten free, as oats may be contaminated with trace amounts of wheat depending on the processing facility or where the crop was grown.)

UNPLUGGED

Brain researchers are discovering a probable relationship between our plugged-in life and the epidemic of "-itis" illnesses. Our natural inflammation balance, which begins in the brain, is wired for daytime brightness and nighttime dimness. The neurohormone melatonin is a powerful inflammation balancer. During sleep – and as lights dim – melatonin increases and helps the brain and body reset into inflammation balance. (See related section, Go Outside and Play, page 180; and Sleep Your Inflammation Away," page 184.)

"Low-fat" = sicker brain. The misguided advice to "eat a low fat diet" is turning out to be one of the sickest medical mantras of the last three decades. We ate less fat, but made up for it by eating more brain and heart-sticky carbs. Not only is a "right fat diet" turning out to be healthier for the heart, it's healthier for the brain. (See related topics low-fat and high-carb, page 122.)

Replacing healthy fats with processed carbs is the diet most likely to inflame the brain. Remember, the brain contains 45 percent of your body's total cholesterol. We are "fatheads" for a smart reason.

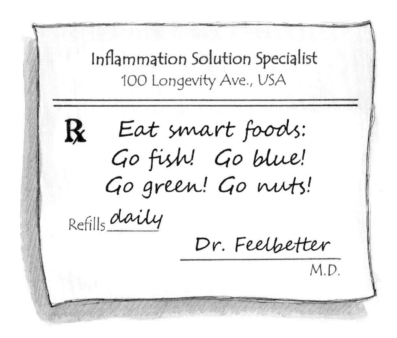

Because it is such a metabolically-active organ, the brain not only uses 20-25 percent of all the oxygen we breathe, it uses 20-25 percent of all the "sugar" we eat. That's why the brain is appropriately called a "carbo hog." Also, because the brain doesn't quickly use fats or proteins for fuel, it is the organ most quickly affected by "low blood sugar," or hypoglycemia. Again, a "right fat" and "right carb" diet, the real food diet, is smartest for the brain.

Fool Your Brain — Fool Your Inflammation

Remember the chip ad, "Bet you can't eat just one!" That's because you can't eat just one. Here's how food chemists fool us and we fool our brain. Food chemists focus on the food-pleasure principle. Just thinking it will taste good triggers your brain's pleasure centers (proven by neuroimaging studies) to plant the idea in your brain: "When I eat this, I will feel good." This inflammation-producing food gimmick works. You eat more and buy more because it is a pleasure food.

Before my health crisis in 1997, I was guilty of the "eat this – feel good" association. Here's how I reshaped my tastes, and my brain. Mentally, I convinced my brain these foods were bad for me, so I didn't eat them. Within four months two amazing taste-shaping changes happened: what I used to crave (i.e., chips), I now shunned. When I caved in and ate a huge helping, my gut would shout "feel bad" signals of pain. So, my gut-brain was reshaped.

Next came the head-brain. When I drove by a fast-food joint (I don't call them restaurants), the visual of the junk food triggered a "pain in the gut" mental image instead of pleasure images. I had mentally changed my perception from "this is a feel-good food" to "this is a feel-bad food." You can do that, too.

The gut-brain's "feel bad" feeling overrides the head-brain's "feel good" pleasure expectations. It's pain over pleasure. It's not worth it. Of course, one of the perks of growing older (and wiser) is that taste buds become more receptive to bitter tastes and less turned on by sweet tastes. Thank you, Mother Nature.

Eat smart foods. Above all other organs, the brain is most affected, for better or worse, by what you eat. As you learned in Chapters Two and Three, smart foods are seafood, blueberries, greens, and nuts.

The Anti-Inflammatory Brain Prescription

What's good for all the other organs is good for the brain:

1. Eat a right-fat diet to feed your "fathead" (see pages 175, 230, 234).

2. Eat a right-carb diet to feed your "carbo hog" (see page 234, 236).

3. Go fish! The same fats that are in fish are the ones nerve tissue needs the most (see page 49).

4. Go nuts (see page 126).

5. Eat "berry good" brain food. Blueberries, I call it "the brain berry," are one of the best neuroprotective antioxidants.

6. Eat Hawaiian astaxanthin. Science shows this supernutrient in seafood is a powerful antioxidant and neuroprotectant.

7. Move! Think "Jog your memory." Movement is one of the best medicines for growing and preserving brain health. Movement:
   - Lowers brain-inflaming sticky stuff.
   - Increases brain-growth neurotropic factor (BGNF), a neurochemical that acts like a fertilizer for brain tissue.

8. Eat less, which can also increase BGNF (see page 143).

9. *Graze* to your brain's content (see page 117).

10. Stay lean (see page 163).

DERMATITIS

Itchy, rough, and uncomfortable skin is one of the most irritating "-itis" illnesses, and one of the most treatable. AGEs, the sticky stuff you learned about on page 45, weaken the collagen proteins, resulting in wrinkles. Inflamed skin is often called "chicken skin" or "alligator skin." Because the skin is exposed to a lot of wear and tear from environmental irritants, it is a set-up for inflammation. Dr. Bill's two-fold anti-inflammatory prescription:

- What you put *into* the skin – anti-inflammatory foods
- What you put *onto* the skin – anti-inflammatory lotions

Feed the skin. The six-S anti-inflammatory diet is just what the dermatologist ordered. Wild Alaskan salmon is a top skin food – think of seafood as skin food – because of the omega-3 oils and the natural anti-inflammatory astaxanthin (see page 87). In fact, astaxanthin has been found to get into the skin and partially protect against sunburn and lessen wrinkles (see page 90). Also, astaxanthin increases the skin's moisture and oil and improves elasticity. These skin-health benefits of astaxanthin are particularly helpful to seniors, since elasticity and moisture content usually lessen with age. Think of astaxanthin as both an internal sunscreen and skin moisturizer. (See astaxanthin, resources, page 267).

Supplement the skin. Science says that omega-3, astaxanthin, and fruit and vegetable supplements all support skin health.

Water the skin. The skin loses a lot of water by exposure to the environment, sweating, and evaporation. Oftentimes the skin also loses some of its natural hydrating and moisturizing ability as we age. Drink at least half an ounce of water per pound of body weight each day. For example, a 140-lb. person should drink 70 ounces, or roughly nine glasses, of water every day.

Moisturize the skin. A skin-health tip I teach in my medical practice, especially for patients with dry skin, is what I call *soak and seal.* After your before-bed bath or shower, gently *pat* (don't rub) the dry, inflamed areas of skin, leaving on a thin layer of water. Cover the slightly-moistened area with a moisturizer to seal in the water to hydrate dry skin. (See related section "Turn down central heat and turn on a vaporizer", page 224.)

Move the skin. Skin massage and total body movement increases blood supply to the skin, which speeds the delivery of more antioxidants and natural anti-inflammatories.

Again, to summarize total-body "-itis" prevention and treatment: eat more fruits, vegetables, and seafood, and go outside and play!

MEASURING YOUR MARKERS

How inflamed are you? Your doctor can measure the inflammation markers in your blood. A marker is an inflammatory biochemical in your blood that goes up, giving you a clue how much excess inflammation is in your body. Over the past decade, enormous technological advances now allow doctors to essentially measure the level of sticky stuff in your blood. Coming soon to the doctor's office near you is a sticky stuff monitor—a gadget that you wear or that allows you to do your own finger stick that monitors the level of sticky stuff biochemicals in your blood and sounds an alarm when they are too high. Another possibility is an app into which you enter

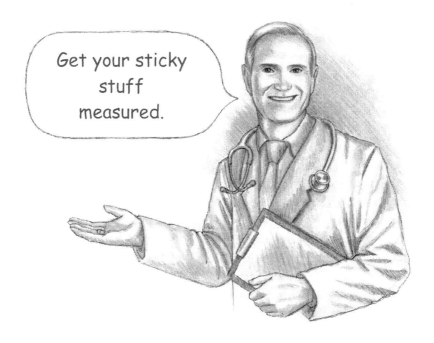

Get your sticky stuff measured.

"cheeseburger," and the tech doctor nags you about how bad the burger is for your body. Stay tuned!

Here are some predictive markers most doctors now measure, depending on what "-itis" you have:

High Sensitivity C-Reactive Protein (HSCRP)

This is the most common test which measures a protein produced by your liver in response to infection, inflammation, or any general over activity of your immune system. It doesn't tell where the inflammation is, only that there is an excess immune response going on *somewhere*. It can go high while fighting the flu, a cold, or even periodontal disease, which is why this test is most meaningful when you don't have a cold, the flu, or any active infection. A chronically elevated CRP may be a clue that you are at risk for cardiovascular disease.

- *Low risk:* less than 1.0 mg/L
- *High risk:* 3-10 mg/L

Hemoglobin A1c (HbA1c)

Whenever your blood sugar is too high for too long, the excess sugar sticks to the hemoglobin in the red blood cells. A high blood level gives a clue that your body is continually pouring out extra insulin to handle excess blood sugar and is also a clue to a person being at risk for developing type II diabetes. (See more about this sticky marker, page 21.)

- *Preferred level:* Less than 6 micro IU/ml

Fasting Insulin

More meaningful than fasting blood sugar, the higher your insulin levels are after fasting, the more you are at risk of developing type II diabetes and other inflammatory illnesses.

- *Preferred level:* Below 15 micro IU/ml

Homocysteine Level

Homocysteine is a sticky amino acid that, if too high, is found to inflame the lining of the arteries. (See related section: Endothelialitis, page 149.) The higher the homocysteine level, the higher a person's risk of developing cardiovascular disease. Some people have a biochemical quirk where they form this sticky stuff during their normal metabolism of foods, especially meat. A high level of homocysteine increases the stickiness of the blood, making it more prone to clots, or coronary thrombosis and stroke. While primarily a genetic quirk, it has also been found in people who have a vitamin B_{12} deficiency.

- *Preferred level:* Below 10 micromol/L

Omega-3 / Omega-6 Blood Levels

As you learned on page 36, both of these fats are healthy, when in balance. Yet, when the omega 6s greatly outnumber the omega-3s, as in the usual SAD (see page 40), the body can be out of balance. A new, but quite informative, test measures the percentage of these fats in the membrane of the red blood cells from a drop of blood. This test gives you the percentage of the important omega fats in your red blood cell membrane and also the ratio of omega-6s-to-omega-3s. Trusted resources for omega measurements:

- OmegaQuant.com
- VitalTEST.com

Healthy level: greater than 8.5 percent of red blood cell membrane fats as omega-3s

Quite often I use this test in my office to motivate patients with low omega-3 levels in their blood to eat seafood or take higher doses of omega-3 fish oil supplements and to give themselves an "oil change" (see page 141).

MEASURING YOUR GENOME

A rapidly evolving science is measuring (either with saliva or blood test) your "genetic tendencies" to certain diseases such as diabetes,

Alzheimer's, cardiovascular disease, cancer, and other inflammatory illnesses. As you learned on page 54, a genetic "tendency" is just that, a tendency. Because we now know that genes only account for a 30 percent influence in certain illnesses (70 percent is lifestyle and diet), if you know you have a genetic risk, you may be motivated to make L.E.A.N. (Lifestyle, Exercise, Attitude, Nutrition) choices to keep that genetic-tendency switch turned off. This sounds like an old Sherlock Holmes dialogue – "It's not our genes that determine our fate, Dr. Watson, it's how we communicate with our genes by the food we eat and the lifestyle we live." (For more information on epigenetics and nutragenetics, see www.PathwayGenomics.com.)

INFLAMMATORY MARKERS FOR CARDIOVASCULAR DISEASE

Oxidized LDL (OxLDL)

LDL cholesterol is not "bad cholesterol." Smart organs, like your brain, need a lot of it. Normal LDL becomes "bad" when it becomes oxidized, meaning it becomes inflamed or "sticky." Oxidized LDL is the stickier cholesterol particle that sticks to the lining of your blood vessels, leading to build-up of plaques. Usually the higher the OxLDL level, the higher the risk of having severe cardiovascular disease.

- *Low:* Less than 45 units/L
- *High:* 45-75 units/L

VAP Cholesterol Test

This blood test measures the number of small-particle cholesterol-carrying molecules, the ones that worm their way into the walls of arteries, contributing to cardiovascular disease. Cholesterol "particle size" is proving to be a more meaningful marker than the usual LDL value.

- Preferred level: under 200 mg/dl

PLAC Test

The PLAC test is a blood test that measures Lp-PLA2, a vascular-specific inflammatory marker that gives a clue that plaque that has accumulated on the wall of an artery is prone to rupture. When arterial walls become inflamed, the enzyme Lp-PLA2 is produced within the plaque. If the amount of Lp-PLA2 is high in the blood, this may indicate that the enzyme is leaking through the plaque and that the plaque is more likely to rupture and release a piece of the plaque into the bloodstream that could cause a clot, leading to a heart attack or stroke. While it's best to prevent the build-up of inflammatory plaque in the first place, if you already have plaque build-up, a high plaque level is just another motivation to make you change and develop your own personal inflammation solution.

Doctors often use the reduction of plaque levels in response to treatment as a way of evaluating results. Statins and fish oil have been shown to lower plaque levels, and the best seems to be statins *plus* omega-3 fish oils.

For the newest lab tests for inflammatory markers, see DrSearsWellnessInstitute.org/resources/inflammation/inflammatory-markers.

WAIST SIZE

In addition to these blood tests, how much flab you can grab gives a clue as to how much inflammation you have. Men with a waist size over 40 inches and women over 35 inches are at increased risk of inflammatory diseases. Your doctor might measure your *waist-hip ratio*. Strive for a ratio below: men: waist/hip: 1:1; women: waist/hip: 0.8:1.

IS CHOLESTEROL IMBALANCE AN INFLAMMATORY ILLNESS?

A classic example of "striking the right balance" is LDL and HDL. LDL, like a ferryboat, carries cholesterol from the liver to tissues such as the brain, adrenal glands (where it is made into hormones like cortisol), sex glands (where it is made into hormones like estrogen and testosterone), and even arterial walls because it is a vital component of all cell membranes all over the body. Its balancing buddy, HDL, is another ferryboat that removes the unneeded and unused cholesterol that LDL deposited and carries it back to the liver so it doesn't pile up in the tissues, especially the walls of the arteries. So it's a question of balance. When LDL becomes too high or too oxidized (sticky) and HDL gets too low, it's this ferryboat imbalance that is "bad" rather than which boat is carrying the cholesterol.

New insights have revealed that perhaps the most beneficial effect of statins is not that they mess with the levels of LDL cholesterol, but rather that they actually act as anti-inflammatories, preventing oxidized (sticky) LDL cholesterol from damaging the arteries. Dr. David Heber, professor of medicine at UCLA, with whom I had the privilege of serving on a medical advisory board, studied red yeast rice, a natural cholesterol-regulating plant used for thousands of years in Chinese medicine, which has received scientific validation as a safer alternative to statins. Studies at The Center for Human Nutrition at UCLA found that red yeast rice lowers sticky LDL in the same, but much safer, way that statins act. Back to Dr. Mother Nature, the most trusted cholesterol-balancer: It's those phytonutrients again – natural biochemicals found in plant foods, called phytosterols (plant, steroid-alcohol), such as found in berries, nuts, grapes, garlic, onions, turmeric, green tea, and olive oil. Seen these foods listed before? Yes, they're in the six-S anti-inflammatory diet. So, for those of you concerned with cholesterol, or for you cholesterol watchers, use the pills-and-skills model by eating the six-S diet, or the L.E.A.N. anti-inflammatory plan, in addition to, or instead of (in consultation with your doctor) cholesterol-lowering prescription medications.

CHAPTER 8

The Inflammation Solution Begins At Birth

While we tend to think that inflammation affects only older people, it really is an illness of all organs at all ages. In fact, new insights reveal that inflammation prevention should start at *birth*. Scientists who study infants are proposing a new theory: how a baby enters the world and how a child is raised can predispose the child to later inflammatory illnesses.

THE MAGICAL MICROBIOME

The inflammation balance of your body is influenced by the microbial balance in your gut. One of the most revealing areas of new inflammation research is that inside our large intestine is a large army of trillions of microbes called the *microbiome* or "bug home." These "good bacteria" naturally inhabit everyone's intestines and, in return for free meals and a warm place to live, they do healthful things for the body. As we grow from birth to adulthood, so do our resident bacteria. A healthy adult may house pounds of hundreds of different species and trillions of bacteria in his or her large intestine. As we learn more about these little critters that live inside us, we realize that if we take care of these little bugs, they do lots of good things for our bodies. And the list of what these little "medicine producers" make is getting longer, including vitamins (such as vitamin K) and healthy fatty acids that provide fuel to help the gut cells lining the colon regrow. They also provide biochemicals that are protective against colon cancer and inflammatory bowel disease. In short, when these bacteria are in balance, they help balance our immune system.

DELIVER BABIES FROM INFLAMMATION

Because of our modern diet and medical practices, could these bountiful little bugs be in danger even before birth? Let's follow the growth of these resident microbes during pregnancy, infancy, and childhood to show you how a baby could be programmed for or against developing inflammatory illnesses later in life.

Mother's microbiome: Better "bugs" build a better immune system for baby. During pregnancy, mother's intestinal and vaginal microbes undergo healthful growth. Mother's birth canal gets populated with health-giving bacteria that she will share with her baby. These beneficial bugs increase in number and healthy function to benefit mother's health and the health of the baby that she will soon give birth to. As Dr. Martin Blasser said in his brilliant book *Missing Microbes:* "These early lactobacilli, which bloomed in mother's vagina during pregnancy, now set up residence and begin to bloom in baby's intestinal tract."

A Tale of Two Births

How a baby is born may affect how healthful a baby's immune system becomes.

Do vaginally-birthed babies have a better immune start? As a vaginally-birthed baby passes through mother's birth canal, baby picks up millions of microscopic microbes, health-promoting bacteria that normally populate the birth canal. These beneficial bugs, called probiotics, then travel into baby's intestines and do healthful things for the growing child, such as help digest foods, make healthy fats, and provide nutrients that help balance the immune system. Like the earliest gut police, they also set-up a foothold in baby's intestinal lining, to crowd out and fight potentially harmful bacteria that are sure to get into baby's gut. These probiotics help protect the vulnerable newborn from the bad bugs that could damage the sensitive gut lining.

Do surgically-birthed babies miss some healthful microbes? The surgically-born baby, which now occurs at a startling rate of 30-40 percent of all births, misses mother's magical microbes as baby passes through the necessarily sterile operating field. Is this probiotic-deprived baby at a higher risk for later developing inflammatory diseases? Some inflammation scientists, such as probiotic expert Dr. Martin Blasser, believe so.

BEST BIRTH "MEDICINE" FOR BABY

Mother's milk, the magical fluid nature perfectly designed for babies, helps build more magical microbes for a healthier gut for our little gal or guy. Put the right bugs in maturing little bowels and healthful things happen. Breast milk helps build better intestinal bacteria that help to digest mother's milk. And like the earliest gut police, these blessed bacteria that are fed by mama's milk also set-up a foothold in the intestinal lining– called *colonization* – to crowd out and fight potential harmful bacteria that are sure to get into baby's gut.

A tale of two milks. For decades, pediatric research has proven that breastfed newborns, especially premature babies that receive their mother's milk (real food, right intestinal bacteria) are not only more likely to grow up smarter, but also have a healthier inflammation balance. Breastfed babies enjoy fewer "-itis" illnesses, such as allergies and eczema, and especially the sometimes fatal newborn intestinal inflammation called *necrotizing enterocolitis*. Here's a bit of baby data: A day's worth (one quart) of mother's milk can nourish baby's gut to grow 10 trillion resident gut bacteria. Add to the formula-fed baby the unhealthful fact that around one-third of infants are now delivered surgically instead of vaginally. Could the type of milk and the route of birth set the infant up for an increased risk of inflammation imbalance later? Research, though still in its infancy, is starting to prove yes.

During breastfeeding, amazing changes start happening inside baby's insides that really emphasize the rightful label "overprotective mother." Consider what the gift of mother's milk contains and, like baby's first immunizations, how it helps protect her precious newborn. As we go through this list, you will understand why in many cultures mother's milk is upgraded to the medically-appropriate label "white blood." Here is a list of some of the immune protectors that mother manufactures and gives baby in her milk.

Immune protection. Mom's "medicine," breast milk, contains millions of white blood cells (germ fighters) and trillions of probiotics. The list of natural immune-strengthening biochemicals is growing, but here are just a few: secretory IgA, lactoferrin, lysozyme, mucin, cytokines, insulin growth factors, interleukins, interferon, tumor necrosis factor, and prostaglandins. A 2014 study from Brigham and Women's Hospital of Harvard Medical School showed that the intestinal microbiome of babies fed their mother's milk recovered more quickly following antibiotic treatment. Pre-term babies, those most vulnerable to infections, really get a big benefit from mother's milk.

Food for the resident bacteria. Like all organisms, you feed these bowel bugs healthy food and they do healthy things for the body. Mother's milk contains a natural prebiotic (food that feeds the gut probiotic bacteria) called oligosaccharides.

Baby's gut lining doesn't leak. A baby's intestines are, shall we say, baby-like. The intestinal lining leaks because the immature lining cells are not close enough to each other. Artificial food and germs and environmental chemicals can "leak" through the gut checkpoints. The last thing you want in a precious newborn baby adapting to our germy world is *leaks* in the lining of the intestines, one of the major entry points for harmful bacteria. Because the intestinal lining of a newborn baby is immature – known as *very permeable* – it's possible that germs and other outside toxins can leak through. Think of the intestinal lining like millions of tiny tiles. It takes a few weeks for the junctions between these tiles to get tighter together and protect against germs leaking through.

Enter Dr. Mother Nature, baby's earliest gastroenterologist. These tiles start closing tighter together (a protective gut phenomenon called "closure") faster in breastfed infants than in formula-fed babies. (Fortunately, by seven to eight months, the intestinal lining of most babies, whether breast- or formula-fed, undergoes protective closure.) And, the breast milk from Dr. Mom is rich in immunoglobulin A (IgA), which is a natural protective sealant that coats the lining of the gut, preventing harmful germs and toxins from leaking through. Also, the natural protective immune biochemicals in mother's milk bind to viruses that may get into the gut and keep them from getting through the lining.

Not so for the formula-fed baby. There is no "white blood" in this man-made milk. No "bugs" at all and that's bad. Because the artificially-fed baby gets artificial baby milk (ABM), baby could be at a higher risk of developing an artificially-acting immune system. Pediatricians correctly dub infant formula ABM. When baby sucks

ABM from a bottle, nothing good happens in the developing little GI tract to help the immune system mature. Feeding babies artificial baby milk at a time in their life when they are most prone to leaky gut, and when the leaky gut is full of bad bacteria, is not a smart inflammation solution.

MOTHER'S MILK: BABY'S FIRST ANTI-INFLAMMATORY FOOD

When mother is exposed to an environmental germ potentially harmful to her baby, Dr. Mom – baby's earliest pharmacist – naturally makes antibodies to this germ and dispenses this "medicine" by way of her milk. Because mother's milk is perfectly formulated, the baby's stomach and upper intestine digest it faster because mother's milk contains natural digestive enzymes, such as lipase for the fat and amylase for the sugars.

Real foods grow real bacteria, which grow real healthy immune systems. The vaginally-birthed, skin-to-skin contact, breastfed baby begins life with a head start in the form of a lowered risk of developing inflammatory diseases. On the other hand, babies who are artificially fed may start life with a "leaky gut," which sets them up for later risks of inflammatory illnesses. With continued mother-baby interaction mommy is, shall we say, sharing the good guys with her little guy. Perhaps this is why mother animals lick their newborns. It seems that nature has worked out the healthiest script for our most precious people, mother and baby. Too bad modern "scientists" don't often follow the script.

THERAPEUTIC BUGS

Probiotics and microbe experts believe that the bacteria that are normally transferred from mother to baby during a vaginal birth and early touch and feeding interactions fill baby's intestines with trillions of tiny bacteria that set the normal bacterial tone for how the gut is supposed to be colonized. Microbe specialists term this early transfer "therapeutically buggy."

TODDLERHOOD: A TALE OF TWO MOMS

Early in my medical practice, I noticed two sets of mothers feeding their toddlers in two different ways. One group fed their children *only real foods*. As a young doctor and young parent, I initially thought these parents were "health food nuts." Using my medical practice as a sort of laboratory, I studied the differences between these "pure kids" of "pure moms" and those who began solid food and toddler feedings from boxes, jars, and cans. What a difference those early feeding habits made! This is why in our pediatric practice, instead of the traditional, boxed starter food, rice cereal, we begin our babies on avocados, bananas, and sweet potatoes around six months of age and salmon at seven months. I advise mothers, when starting solid foods, to "think outside the box." (See AskDrSears.com/solidfoods.)

In general, the real-food eating kids weren't sick as often. When these pure kids of pure moms went to birthday parties, and preschool, of course these normal kids tried the junk food. But when they did, they felt what they called "yucky tummy." Called *metabolic programming*, the real-food parents had programmed their child's gut: "You eat real foods, you feel real good."

IS SCHOOL HAZARDOUS TO A CHILD'S HEALTH?

The final insult happens when the child goes to school. If the good bugs in the gut could talk, they would say, "Get ready for the pains in the gut that are so common to school children." Gut microbial health, in a nutshell, is that good bugs thrive on good food, and bad bugs thrive on bad food.

The child who enjoyed the immune protection of mother's milk and a real food diet in those early years starts school with an inflammation-balance head start. In my medical practice, I notice these children are usually healthier during the school years.

The child who begins school with a shaky immune start is more likely to be sick more often at school, for three reasons:

- Exposed to more germs the children "share."
- Exposed to more immune-system-weakening foods.
- Sits more than moves.

New insights reveal that many of the "Ds" that label school kids may have their root cause in inflammation.

Old approach: Child enters doctor's office, referred by school or therapist for treatment of a "D": (Attention Deficit/Hyperactivity Disorder [ADHD], Obsessive Compulsive Disorder [OCD], Borderline Personality Disorder [BPD], and so on). Hurried doctor thinks:

- "What 'D' box do I put this child in?"
- "What D-drug do I put this child on?
- Next patient!

New approach: Based on new research, before drugging the child for a D, try the anti-inflammatory six-S diet and get the child moving. In other words, try physiological before pharmacological (skills before pills) treatment. As Dr. Mom prescribed: Eat more fruits and vegetables and go outside and play!

For informative resources on making health and nutrition changes in schools see: *The Nutrition Detectives Program* and *ABC for Fitness (Activity Bursts in the Classroom)* by David Katz, M.D.

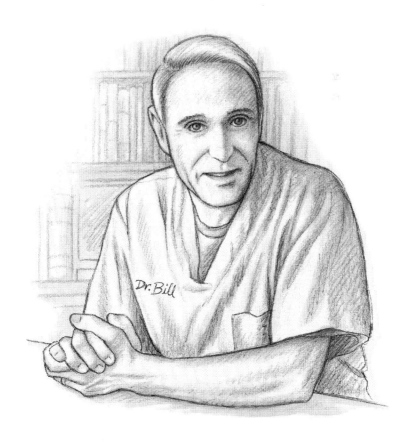

DO CHILDREN GET TOO MANY PILLS?

Other things go on to perhaps set the child up for adult inflammatory diseases. While modern antibiotics have been healthy and lifesaving, there is a growing concern among pediatricians that their overuse may have harmed the normal intestinal bacteria, sort of like going into a battle and killing the bad guys – the germs – but also, unfortunately, killing the good guys that are there for healthful reasons. Could this early imbalance of bacteria be setting a child up for inflammation imbalances as an adult? More and more doctors are thinking yes. This concern has prompted more doctors to exercise more caution in prescribing too many antibiotics, especially drugs that are too strong for too long. We also try to "match the drug to the bug," prescribing a milder antibiotic instead of a "broad spectrum" antibiotic, whenever possible.

CHILDHOOD INFLAMMATION SOLUTIONS

By improving birthing practices, enhancing breastfeeding, and feeding kids real food, we can give children a good gut start toward reducing the risk of growing up to be adults with "-itis" illnesses. Here's how:

Inflammation Solution #1: Have a Healthy Pregnancy and Birth

To increase your opportunity to have a healthy, natural birth, here's my prescription: Read *The Healthy Pregnancy Book* (Little Brown, 2013). This is presently the only pregnancy book coauthored by an obstetrician, certified midwife / Ph.D., pediatrician, R.N. and mother of eight. By following the healthy pregnancy plan, you are more likely to start mother and baby off on a life at lower risk for inflammation.

Inflammation Solution #2: Breastfeed

I have a dream. Realizing that the government healthcare system funding is backwards – spending tons of money on treatment instead of prevention – if I were Surgeon General for a day, here's what I would do:

- Provide financial incentives for more mothers to breastfeed more often and for many more months.

- Provide every first-time mother with a professional lactation consultant before and immediately after birth. Doctor's orders!

- Educate birth and postpartum attendants – and all baby care professionals – to be more positive about breastfeeding and avoid discouraging words, such as "…in case you don't have enough milk…"

- Play show and tell. Educate expectant and new mothers on how much better their milk is than ABM and how, if you breastfeed your baby, you give your baby a head start on developing a healthy immune system. On the other hand, starting a baby off with ABM runs the risk of baby later growing an artificial immune system.

- Provide financial incentives for workplaces to have comfortable *lactation lounges* that make breastfeeding and working friendlier. It's noteworthy that some of the smartest companies are encouraging mothers to continue breastfeeding after returning to work. Why? Money! Breastfeeding mothers tend to miss fewer days of work because their infants aren't sick as often.

- Fund and provide a safe system for donor breast milk in case there are medical or family situations whereby baby is unable to be fed by mother's milk.

Since science shows breastfed babies suffer fewer "-itis" illnesses and the incidence of just about every disease is less in breastfed babies, imagine the billions of dollars in healthcare cost savings. Currently, the government and insurance companies pay for treatment instead of prevention. They pay for pills rather than teaching skills. If only kids could vote!

Inflammation Solution #3: Shape Young Tastes

Especially in those early years, serve infants and children a *real food diet*. Our inflammation prescription: MYOBF – make your own baby food. The foods your child's tastes and intestinal lining gets used to (metabolic programming) are more likely to set the child up for life-long healthy eating habits.

Inflammation Solution #4: Eat Prebiotic Foods

The gold standard of prebiotics (foods that help healthy bacteria thrive) is breast milk. Could it be that when we feed the normal gut bacteria junk food we get back junk gut health? The bad bugs in the gut thrive on bad adult behavior such as drinking too much sweetened beverages and alcohol and eating too little fiber. Perhaps we need to extend one of the oldest gut teachings from "we are what we eat" to "we are what the bugs in our bowels eat."

"Take probiotics" is a new supplement suggestion coming to the healthcare stores, even doctors' offices, near you. Add to this somewhat-science-supported advice, "Eat prebiotics." Prebiotics are foods that help the best bowel bugs thrive. Just like the truism "your body is as only as healthy as the food you feed it" add "the bugs in our bodies are only as healthy as the food we feed them." Best bowel-bug foods are:

- Jerusalem artichokes
- Chicory root
- Onions
- Garlic
- Leeks
- Bananas
- Tomatoes
- Spinach
- Oatmeal
- Barley
- Flax seed
- Legumes

I believe if my microbiome could talk, it would shout: "We love the six-S diet!"

Inflammation Solution #5: Make Schools More Healthy

There is an epidemic of "Ds" in schools: Attention Deficit Disorder (ADD), ADHD, and so on. Let me add two more school-related "Ds": NDD (Nutrition Deficit Disorder) and MDD (Movement Deficit Disorder). Serve children junk food and you get junk learning and behavior. When recess was taken out of school activities, Ritalin dosages went up. Any correlation? Read these resources for feeding little brains for better learning and behavior:

- *The Healthiest Kid in the Neighborhood: Ten Ways to Get Your Family on the Right Nutritional track* by William, Martha, James, and Robert Sears. 2008, Little, Brown and Company.

- *The NDD Book: How Nutrition Deficit Disorder Affects Your Child's Learning, Behavior, and Health, and What You Can Do About It – Without Drugs* by William Sears. 2009, Little, Brown and Company.

Inflammation Solution #6: Go Outside and Play

Dr. Mom's medical prescription, "Eat more fruits and vegetables and go outside and play" has never been timelier. (See why, pages 29 and 180.) For good veggie tips, read: *Vegetable Soup/The Fruit Bowl* by Susan Smith Jones and Dianne Warren, 2014, Oasis Publishing. (www.SusanSmithJones.com)

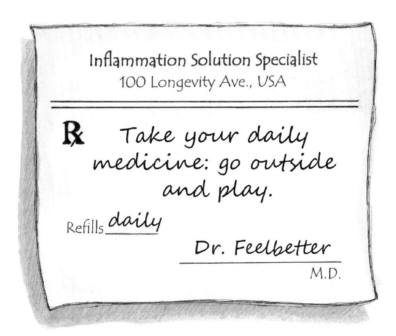

Inflammation Solution Specialist
100 Longevity Ave., USA

℞ Take your daily medicine: go outside and play.

Refills _daily_

Dr. Feelbetter

M.D.

Chapter 9

A Summary: Dr. Bill's Anti-inflammatory Prescription. Read It, Do It, Feel It!

How diligently you do these ten changes will determine how quickly you feel better. You may decide to take the *slow track* and make only one or two major changes each week, easing into the whole plan over several months. That's okay. You know what's best for you. Your goal: to feel an *inflammation transformation* that works and lasts.

My recommendations: Take the *fast track*. Make all ten changes. Give it a 6-week trial. The fast track helps you feel the difference sooner, providing a more lasting motivation to continue. By reprogramming your body over a couple months, you go from: "Don't like it, but must do it," to "Like it a little," to "Like it a lot," and finally to "*Crave it.*" We want you to get that WOW feeling: "I feel so much better, I'll never go back!"

Medically speaking, this is called *metabolic programming*. By reshaping your tastes and caring for your body the way it was meant to be cared for, you turn on some inner switch inside that prompts you: This is the way you are meant to live. You are resetting your body into inflammation balance. Called the *wisdom of the body*, wherever that inside switch is turned on, if it could talk, it would say: "Because you are treating me so well, I will treat you well." You are well on your way to

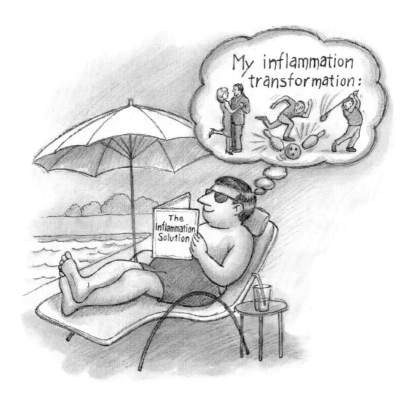

achieving your health wish: Everything works and nothing hurts. Let's get started:

TEN STEPS TOWARD ENJOYING YOUR PERSONAL INFLAMMATION TRANSFORMATION

1. Make Health Your Hobby

Top on most doctors' wish list is a model of self-care we call *personalized medicine*, formulating an inflammation-balancing plan that fits your individual body. However, the economic realities of healthcare reform prevent most doctors from spending the extra patient time to make this happen. Solution: formulate your own personal health plan and use your doctor as a trusted consultant.

Take a health trip. Take a week or weekend off. Rest and meditate on your health goals.

- I will make health my hobby.
- I will make The Inflammation Solution Program my priority.
- I will, as much as possible, adjust my L.E.A.N. (see page 34) to fit this priority.

During your health sabbatical, read this book cover-to-cover, highlighting the health changes you most need to make.

Program your mind to do it and feel it. As you are reading and meditating on this program you are about to begin, imagine your inflammation transformation happening. Picture yourself with more physical energy, greater mental clarity, painless living, and doing more activities (dancing, swinging a golf club) that your mind wants to do, but your body hurts too much to do.

Food for thought? This could be you!

2. Make Your Health Progress Chart

Journal your plan and your progress. Note *what you've done* and *how you now feel*. If you have a family, let them know what you are doing and why. My close friend, Harry, called a family meeting and announced, "As you all know, Dad hasn't been feeling well and taking care of himself. You will be happy to know, because I love you and want to be a committed dad and granddad; I'm starting a total health-plan makeover. I want not only to be at the weddings of my grandchildren, I want to dance at them." What a health role model

Harry became to his family, and what a lasting inheritance he will leave them.

Schedule a check-up with your healthcare provider.

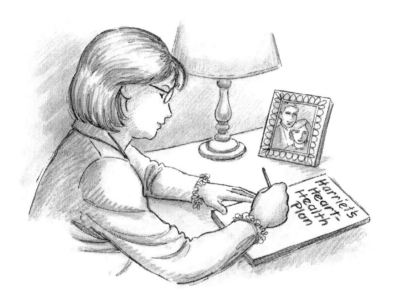

Health	Before changes	After changes
• Inflammatory markers (page 238)		
• Anti-inflammatory medications		
• Waist size		
• Joint pain		
• Intestinal upsets		
• Whatever hurts and doesn't work		

3. Do a Home Makeover

- Get junk food out; out of sight equals out of mouth. Remove all foods that contain chemical sticky stuff. (See lists on pages 99 and 108.)
- A home gym (see page 217).
- If possible, place desk near a window.
- Compile your home Inflammation Solution library. (See resources, page 267.)

3. Enjoy the Sipping Solution 5 Days a Week (page 57)

4. Follow the Six-S Anti-inflammatory Diet 5 Days a Week (page 39)

- Give yourself an oil change (see page 141).
- Eat The Inflammation Solution way (see page 39).

5. Graze On Good Foods

- Follow the rule of twos (see page 117).
- Use chopsticks instead of a fork (see page 118).
- Snack smart (see page 58).

6. Move More

- Commit to 30-60 minutes of strenuous exercise each day, 5-6 days a week (see page 145).
- Do isometric, anytime /anywhere exercises at least *20 minutes daily* (see page 217).
- Do joint-specific movements daily, e.g., swimming, knee-pumping (see page 199 – 221).

No excuses please! If you think, "But I don't have time to exercise an hour a day," then you're thinking that you would rather spend more time hurting!

Make a list of all those moments you could be moving instead of sitting, such as:

- Parking farther away and walking a few blocks to your work.
- Taking stairs instead of escalators or elevators (be aware that stair-stepping is often not friendly to knee joints).
- While at your desk, do isometrics (see page 217).
- While standing, do isometrics (see page 217).
- Walk while you talk on the phone.
- Correspond less by email, and do more *walk while you talk*. Instead of a long email, set up a call time. I tell my emailers, "I think and communicate better by phone, please call me at…" One week I kept a log and realized I could walk an extra half-hour a day by this move more, sit less strategy.

7. Stress Less

- Put together your own stressbuster strategies and meditation habits (see page 180).
- Keep focusing on how much better you will soon feel.

8. Sleep Soundly (See sleep tips, page 184.)

9. Enjoy the Helper's High

Once you feel it, you will want to share it. Play show and tell. When your friends and family see your transformation, tell them how you did it,

- *Share* your plan with others: spouse, friends
- *Partner* with a hurting friend. Motivate and hold each other accountable.
- *Serve*: Volunteer
- *Teach*: Become a Dr. Sears Certified Health Coach (see page 269)

You're in rehab. I love the term "rehab," which is usually a very healthy title: remaking your habits – for the better. Not that I am advising you "-itis" sufferers to announce to your love ones, "I'm in rehab," but you are. By following The Inflammation Solution, you are embarking on an inflammation transformation, changing your habits from those that cause you to feel bad to those that help you feel good.

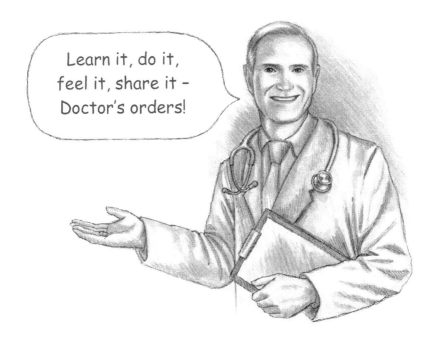

Learn it, do it, feel it, share it – Doctor's orders!

YOUR INFLAMMATION SOLUTION CHECKLIST

Post this reminder list on your washbasin mirror:

- ✓ Eat only inflammation solution foods (or at least 90/10).
- ✓ Eat more seafood, less meat.
- ✓ Graze according to the rule of twos.
- ✓ Use chopsticks.
- ✓ Sip on a smoothie for breakfast, snacks and lunch.
- ✓ Eat seafood for dinner 3-4 evenings a week.
- ✓ Eat more inflammation-balancing oils.
- ✓ Eat salad before your biggest meal of the day.
- ✓ Eat more plant-based and less animal-based foods.
- ✓ Move more, sit less.
- ✓ Stand smart, don't lock knees.
- ✓ Talk while you walk; more phone, less email.
- ✓ Do isometrics; anytime, anywhere exercises.
- ✓ Take several deep breaths hourly.
- ✓ Meditate, nature walks and views.
- ✓ Did you journal today?

RESOURCES

GENERAL - BOOKS

Prime-Time Health: A Scientifically Proven Plan for Feeling Young and Living Longer, William and Martha Sears, Little Brown, 2010. Also available on DVD from DrSearsWellnessInstitute.org.

The N.D.D. Book: How Nutrition Deficit Disorder Affects Your Child's Learning, Behavior and Health and What You Can Do About it – Without Drugs, William Sears, Little Brown, 2009

The Omega-3 Effect: Everything You Need to Know About the Supernutrient for Living Longer, Healthier, and Happier, William Sears, Little Brown, 2012

Natural Astaxanthin: Hawaii's Supernutrient, by William Sears, M.D. 2015

The Hawaiian Spirulina Equation, Bob Capelli, 2014.

GENERAL - WEBSITES

See DrSearsWellnessInstitute.org/resources/inflammation for updates on inflammation solutions and personal testimonies.

Get a free copy of *Natural Astaxanthin: Hawaii's Supernutrient* from http://www.nutrex-hawaii.com

Visit Vitalchoice.com to subscribe to my favorite seafood source and newsletter.

Visit JuicePlus.com for information on the most scientifically researched fruit and vegetable concentrate.

USDA National Nutrient Database: http://ndb.nal.usda.gov

Learn how to become a Dr. Sears Certified Health Coach at DrSearsWellnessInstitute.org.

CHAPTER 1: WHAT "-ITIS" IS IN YOUR BODY?

1. http://www.cdc.gov/nchs/fastats/arthritis.htm

2. http://www.cdc.gov/features/jointpain/index.html

3. William Sears and Martha Sears, *Prime-Time Health: A Scientifically Proven Plan for Feeling Young and Living Longer*, Little, Brown, 2010.

4. William Sears with James Sears, *The Omega-3 Effect: Everything You Need to Know About the Supernutrient for Living Longer, Healthier, and Happier*, Little, Brown, 2012.

5. *Natural Astaxanthin – Hawaii's Supernutrient* , by Dr. William Sears, M.D. 2015.

6. Jason Theodosakis, *The Arthritis Cure*, St. Martin's Press, 2004.

7. Osei, K., et al. Is Glycosylated Hemoglobin A1c a Surrogate for Metabolic Syndrome in Nondiabetic, First-Degree Relatives of African-American Patients with Type 2 Diabetes? *Journal of Clinical Endocrinology Metabolism* (2003); 88:4596-4601

8. Khaw K-T, Wareham, N., Luben, R., Bingham, S., Oakes, S., Welch, A., et al. Glycosylated haemoglobin, diabetes and mortality in men in Norfolk cohort of European Prospective Investigation of Cancer and Nutrition (EPIC-Norfolk). *BMJ* (2001); 322:15-18

9. William Sears, *The Sears' L.E.A.N. Program* (See DrSearsWellnessInstitute.org)

CHAPTER 2: EAT ANTI-INFLAMMATORY FOODS

1. William Sears, Resource #1, *Prime-Time Health*, Little Brown, 2010.

2. Walter Cannon, *The Wisdom of the Body*, W. W. Norton and Company, 1963.

3. Jorn Dyerberg, personal communication, March 2011.

4. Maroon, J.C., and Bost, J.W. Omega-3 fatty acids (fish oil) as an anti-inflammatory: An alternative to nonsteroidal anti-inflammatory drugs for discogenic pain. *Surgical Neurology* (2006); 65:326-331.

5. Damsgaard, C.T., Lauritzen, L., Kjaer, T.M., et al. Fish oil supplementation modulates immune function in healthy infants. *Journal of Nutrition* (2007); 137:1031-1036.

6. Schubert, R., Kitz, R., Beerman, C., et al, Effect of n-3 polyunsaturated fatty acids in asthma after low-dose allergen challenge. *International Archives of Allergy and Immunology* (2009); 148:321-329.

7. Pascoe, M.C., et al., What you eat is what you are – a role for polyunsaturated fatty acids in neuroinflammation-induced depression. *Clinical Nutrition* (2011); 30:407-15.

8. Akinkuolie, A.O., Ngwa, J.S., Meigs, J.B. et al., Omega-3 polyunsaturated fatty acid and insulin sensitivity: A meta-analysis of randomized controlled trials. *Clinical Nutrition* (2011); 30:702-707.

9. Kaye, E.K. n-3 fatty acid intake and periodontal disease, *Journal of the American Dietetic Association* (2010); 110:1650-1652. See also A.Z. Naqvi, C. Buettner, R.S. Phillips et al., n-3 fatty acids and periodontitis in U.S. adults. *Journal of the American Dietetic Association* (2010); 110:1669-1675.

10. Hasturk, H., Kantarci, A., Goguet-Surmenian, E., et al., Resolvin E1 regulates inflammation at the cellular and tissue level and restores tissue homeostatis in vivo. *Journal of Immunology* (2007); 179:7021-7029.

11. Koch, C., Dölle, S., Metzger, M., et al., Docosahexaenoic acid (DHA) supplementation in atopic eczema: A randomized, double-blind, controlled trial. *British Journal of Dermatology* (2008); 158: 786-792.

12. Alm, B., Aberg, N., Erdes, L., et al., Early introduction of fish decreases the risk of eczema in infants. *Archives of Disease in Childhood* (2009); 94:11-15;

13. Furuhjelm, C., Warstedt, K., Larsson, J., et al., Fish oil supplementation in pregnancy and lactation may decrease the risk of infant allergy. *Acta Paediatrica* (2009); 98:1461-1467.

14. Houston, M., et al. Nonpharmacologic treatment of dyslipidemia. *Progress in Cardiovascular Disease* (2009); 52:61-94.

15. Roche, H.M., and Gibney, M.J. Effect of long chain n-3 polyunsaturated fatty acids on fasting and postprandial triacylglycerol metabolism. *American Journal of Clinical Nutrition* (2000); 71: 2325-2375.

16. Griffin, M. D., Sanders, T.A., Davies, I.G., et al., Effects of altering the ratio of dietary n-6 to n-3 fatty acids on insulin sensitivity, lipoprotein size, and postprandial lipemia in men and postmenopausal women aged 45-70 y: The OPTILIP study. *American Journal of Clinical Nutrition* (2005); 84:1290-1298.

17. Parra, D., Ramel, A., Bandarra, N. et al., A diet rich in long-chain omega-3 fatty acids modulates satiety in overweight and obese volunteers during weight loss. *Appetite* (2008); 51:676-680.

18. Ridker, P.M., et al., Rouvastatin to prevent vascular events in men and women with elevated C-reactive protein. *New England Journal of Medicine* (2008); November 9.

19. Chandra, G., and Aggarwal, B. "Spicing up" the immune system by curcumin. *Journal of Immunology* (2007); 27:19-34.

20. Kang, W.S., et al., Anti-thrombotic activities of green tea catechins and (-) epigallo catechin gallate. *Thrombosis Research* (1999); 96:229-237.

21. Nakagawa, T., et al., Protective activity of green tea against free radical and glucose-mediated protein damage. *Journal of Agricultural and Food Chemistry* (2002); 8:2418-22.

22. Klipstein-Grobusch, K., et al., Serum carotenoids and atherosclerosis: The Rotterdam Study. *Atherosclerosis* (2000); 148:49-56.

23. Fukugawa, N.K., et al., Effects of age on body composition and resting metabolic rate. *American Journal of Physiology* (1990); 259: E 233-8.

24. Kim, J.Y., et al., Effects of lycopene supplementation on oxidative stress and markers of endothelial function in healthy men. *Atherosclerosis* (2011); 215:189-95.

25. Douglas-Escobar, M., et al., Effects of intestinal microbial ecology on the developing brain. *JAMA Pediatrics* (2013); 167:374-79.

26. Serhan, C.N. How DHA Tames Inflammation. *FASEB Journal* (2013); 2573-83

27. Harris, D., et al., Cigarette smoking renders LDL susceptible to perioxidative modification and enhanced metabolism by macrophages. *Atherosclerosis* (1989); 79:245-252.

28. Sano, J., et al., Effects of green tea intake on the development of coronary artery disease. *Circulation Journal* (2004); 68:665-670.

29. Van de lest, C.H., et al., Loading-induced changes on synovial fluid affect cartilage metabolism. *Biorheology* (2000); 37:45-55.

30. Wattanathorn, J., et al., Pipersine, the potential functional food for mood and cognitive disorders. *Food Chemistry Toxicology* (2008); 46:3106-10.

31. Abascal, K., et al., The medicinal uses of cinnamon. *Integrative Medicine* (2010); 9:29-32.

32. Hlebowitz, J., et al., Effect of cinnamon on postprandial blood glucose. *American Journal of Clinical Nutrition* (2007); 85:1552-(?).

33. Khan, A., et al., Cinnamon improves glucose and lipids of people with type 2 diabetes. *Diabetes Care* (2003); 26:3215-3218.

34. Bland, J., et al., Clinical Pearls from the 11th International Symposium on Functional Medicine. *Integrative Medicine* (2004); 5:32-36.

35. Soni, K.B., et al., Effect of oral curcumin administration on serum peroxides and cholesterol levels in human volunteers. *Indian Journal of Physiology and Pharmacology* (1992); 36: 273-275.

36. Chainani-Woo, N. Safety and anti-inflammatory activity of curcumin: A component of turmeric (curcuma wonga). *Journal of Alternative and Complimentary Medicine* (2003); 9: 161-168.

37. Park, J., et al. Anti-carcinogenic properties of curcumin on colorectal cancer. *World Journal of Gastrointestinal Oncology* 2010; 2(4): 169-176.

38. Merle, B.M., et al. High concentrations of plasma n3 fatty acids are associated with decreased risk for late age-related macular degeneration. *Journal of Nutrition.* 2013 Apr; 143(4):505-11.

39. Shah, B.H., et al., Inhibitory effect of curcumin, a food spice from turmeric, on platelet-activating factor and arachnidonic acid mediated platelet aggregation through inhibition of thromboxane formation in Ca signaling. *Biochemical Pharmacology* (1999); 58:1167-1172.

40. Anderson, R., et al., Cinnamon. *Diabetic Care* (2003); 26:3215-3218.

41. Aggarwal, B.B. *Healing Spices: How To Use 50 Everyday and Exotic Spices to Boost Health and Beat Disease*, Sterling Publishing, New York, 2011.

42. Yang, F., et al. Curcumin Inhibits Formation of Amyloid β Oligomers and Fibrils, Binds Plaques, and Reduces Amyloid *in Vivo.* February 18, 2005. *The Journal of Biological Chemistry*, 280, 5892-5901

43. Breithaupt-Frogler, K., et al., Protective effect of chronic garlic intake on elastic properties of aorta in the elderly. *Circulation* (1997); 96:2649-2655.

44. Fleischaur, A.T., et al., Garlic consumption and cancer prevention: meta-analysis of colorectal and stomach cancers. *American Journal of Clinical Nutrition* (2000); 72:147-52.

45. Chan, C.H.,et al., Antioxidative and anti-inflammatory neuroprotective effects of astaxanthin and canthaxanthin in nerve growth factor differentiated PC12 cells. *Journal of Food Science* (2009); 74(7): H225-31.

46. Fassett, R.G., et al., Astaxanthin versus placebo on arterial stiffness, oxidative stress, and inflammation in renal transplant patients: A randomized, controlled trial. *BMC Nephrology* (2008); 9:17.

47. Iwamoto, T., et al., Inhibition of low-density lipoprotein oxidation by astaxanthin. *Journal of Atherosclerosis and Thrombosis.* (2000); 7(4):216-22.

48. Izumi-Nagai, K., et al., Inhibition of choroidal neovascularization with an anti-inflammatory carotenoid astaxanthin. *Investigative Opthalmology and Visual Science.* (2008); 49(4):1679-85.

49. Lee, D.H., et al., Astaxanthin protects against MPTP/MPP+-induced mitochondrial dysfunction and ROS production in vivo and in vitro. *Food and Chemical Toxicology.* (2011); 49(1):271-80.

50. Miyawaki, H., et al., Effects of astaxanthin on human blood rheology. *Journal of Clinical Biochemistry and Nutrition* (2008); 43(2):9-74.

51. Nakagawa, K., et al., Anti-oxidant effect of astaxanthin on phospholipid peroxidation in human erythrocytes. *British Journal of Nutrition*, (2011); 105(11):1563-71.

52. Palozza, P., et al., Growth-inhibiting effects of the astaxanthin-rich haematococcus pluvialis in human colon cancer cells. *Cancer Letters* (2009); 283(1):108-17.

53. Park, J.S., et al., Astaxanthin decreased oxidative stress and inflammation and enhanced immune response in humans. *Nutrition and Metabolism* (2010); March 5; 7:18.

54. Pashkow, F.J., et al. Astaxanthin: A novel potential treatment for oxidative stress and inflammation and cardiovascular disease. *The American Journal of Cardiology* (2008); 101(10a):58d-68d.

55. Sun, Z., et al. Protective actions of microalgae against endogenous and exogenous AGEs in human retinal pigment epithelial cells. *Food and Function* (2011); 2(5):251-8.

56. Wang, H.Q., et al. Astaxanthin upregulates heme oxygenase-1 expression through ERK 1/2 pathway and its protective effect against beta-amyloid-induced cytotoxicity in SH-SY5Y cells. *Brain Research* (2010); 1360:159-67.

57. Yoshida H., et al. Administration of Natural Astaxanthin increases serum HDL-cholesterol and adiponectin in subjects with mild hyperlipidemia. *Atherosclerosis* (2010); 209:520-3.

58. Higuera-Ciapara, I., Felix-Valenzuela, L., Goycoolea, F.M. Astaxanthin: A review of its chemistry and applications. *Critical Reviews in Food Science and Nutrition.* (2006); 46(2):185-96.

59. Yasui, Y., Hosokawa, M., Miyashita, K., Tanaka, T. Dietary astaxanthin inhibits colitis and colitis-associated colon carcinogenesis in mice via modulation of the inflammatory cytokines. *Chemico-Biological Interactions* (2011); Aug 15; 193(1):79-87.

60. Liu, X., Osawa, T. Astaxanthin protects neuronal cells against oxidative damage and is a potent candidate for brain food. *Forum of Nutrition.* (2009); 61:129-35.

61. Tominaga, K., Hongo, N., Karato, M., Yamashita, E. Cosmetic benefits of astaxanthin on human subjects. *Acta Biochimica Polonica.* (2012); 59(1):43-7.

62. Chew, B.P., Park, J.S. Carotenoid action on the immune response. *Journal of Nutrition.* (2004); Jan: 134(1): 257S-61S.

63. Ye, Q., Huang, B., Zhang, X., Zhu, Y., Chen, X. Astaxanthin protects against MPP+-induced oxidative stress in PC12 cells via the HO-1/NOX2 axis. *BMC Neuroscience* (2012); Dec 29, 13(1):156.

64. Kiko, T., Nakagawa, K., Satoh, A., et al., Amyloid beta levels in human red blood cells. *PLoS One* (2012); 7(11):e49620.

65. Pabon, M.M., et al. A spirulina-enhanced diet provides neuroprotection in an α-synuclein model of Parkinson's disease. *PLoS One* 2012;7(9):e45256.

66. Capelli, B. *The Hawaiian Spirulina Equation.* 2014.

67. Cui, X., et al., Suppression of DNA damage in human peripheral blood lymphocytes by a juice concentrate: A randomized double-blind, placebo-controlled trial. *Molecular Nutrition and Food Research* (2012); 56: 1-5.

68. Jin, Y., Cui, X., et al. Systemic inflammatory load in humans is suppressed by consumption of two formulations of dried encapsulated juice concentrate. *Molecular Nutrition and Food Research* (2010); 54:1506-14.

69. Chapple, I.L., et al. Adjunctive daily supplementation with encapsulated fruit, vegetable and berry juice powder concentrates and clinical periodontal outcomes: a double-blind RCT. *Journal of Clinical Periodontology* (2012); 39:62-72.

70. Canas, J.A., et al. Insulin resistance and adiposity in relation to serum beta-carotene levels. *Journal of Pediatrics* (2012); 161(1):58-64.

71. Novembrino, C., et al. Effects of encapsulated fruit and vegetable juice powder concentrate on oxidative status in heavy smokers. *Journal of the American College of Nutrition* (2011); 30:49-56.

72. Bamonti, F., et al. An encapsulated juice powder concentrate improves markers of pulmonary function and cardiovascular risk factors in heavy smokers. *Journal of the American College of Nutrition* (2013); 32(1):18-25.

73. Lamprecht, M., Obermayer, G., Steinbauer, K., et al., Supplementation with a juice powder concentrate and exercise decrease oxidation and inflammation, and improve the microcirculation in obese women: randomized controlled trial data. *British Journal of Nutrition* (2013); http://www.ncbi.nlm.nih.gov/pubmed/23075557.

74. Kiefer, et al., Supplementation with mixed fruit and vegetable juice concentrated increased serum antioxidants and folate in healthy adults. *Journal of the American College of Nutrition* (2004); 23:205-211.

75. Nantz, M., et al. Immunity and antioxidant capacity in humans is enhanced by consumption of a dried, encapsulated fruit and vegetable juice concentrate. *Journal of Nutrition* (2006); 136:2606-2610.

76. Lamprecht M., Oettl K., Schwaberger G., et al. Protein modification responds to exercise intensity and antioxidant supplementation. *Medicine and Science in Sports and Exercise* (2009); 41:155-163.

77. Goldfarb A.H., Garten R.S., Cho C., et al. Effects of a fruit/berry/vegetable supplement on muscle function and oxidative stress. *Medicine and Science in Sports and Exercise* (2011); 43:501-8.

78. Bellavia, A., et al. Fruit and vegetable consumption and all-cause mortality: a dose-response analysis. *American Journal of Clinical Nutrition.* 2013 98: 454-9.

79. Reddy, B.S., et al. Chemoprevention of Colon Carcinogenesis by Dietary Curcumin, a Naturally Occurring Plant Phenolic Compound. *Cancer Research* (1995); 55: 259-266.

80. Panunzio M.F., et al. Supplementation with a fruit and vegetable concentrate decreases plasma homocysteine levels in a dietary controlled trial. *Nutrition Research* (2003); 23(9):1221-8.

81. Samman, S., et al. A mixed fruit and vegetable concentrate increases plasma antioxidant vitamins and folate and lowers plasma homocysteine in men. *Journal of Nutrition.* (2003); 133(7):2188-93.

82. Lamprecht, M., et al. Several indicators of oxidative stress, immunity, and illness improved in trained men consuming an encapsulated juice powder concentrate for 28 weeks. *Journal of Nutrition.* (2007) Dec;137(12):2737-41.

83. Plotnick, G.D., et al. Effect of supplemental phytonutrients on impairment of the flow-mediated brachial artery vasoactivity after a single high-fat meal. *Journal of the American College of Cardiology.* 2003 May 21;41(10):1744-9.

84. Esfahani, A., et al. Health effects of mixed fruit and vegetable concentrates: a systematic review of the clinical interventions. *Journal of the American College of Nutrition* 2011;30(5):285-294.

85. Bloomer, R.J., et al. Oxidative stress response to aerobic exercise: comparison of antioxidant supplements. *Medicine and Science in Sports and Exercise.* 2006 Jun;38(6):1098-105.

86. Kawashima, A., et al. Four week supplementation with mixed fruit and vegetable juice concentrates increased protective serum antioxidants and folate and decreased plasma homocysteine in Japanese subjects. *Asia Pacific Journal of Clinical Nutrition.* 2007;16(3):411-21.

87. Holick, M. *The Vitamin D Solution: A 3-Step Strategy to Cure Our Most Common Health Problems.* Hudson Street Press, 2010.

88. Mason, C., et al. Vitamin D3 supplementation during weight loss: a double-blind randomized controlled trial. *American Journal of Clinical Nutrition.* 2014 May; 99(5):1015-25.

89. Kuriyama, S., et al. Green tea consumption and mortality due to cardiovascular disease, cancer and all causes in Japan: The OHSAKI Study. *JAMA* 2000; 296:1255-65.

CHAPTER 3: TWELVE SIMPLE WAYS TO EAT THE ANTI-INFLAMMATORY WAY

1. P.M. Luhrman, et al., Changes in resting metabolic rate in an elderly German population: cross-sectional and longitudinal data. *Journal of Nutrition and Healthy Aging* (2010); 14:232-36.

2. Erbad, et al. Effectiveness of Moderate Green Tea Consumption on Anti-Oxidative Status and Plasma Lipid Profile in Humans. *Journal of Nutritional Biochemistry* (2005) 16:144-149.

3. Unno, T., et al. Effect of Tea Catechins on Post-Prandial Plasma Lipid Responses in Human Subjects. *British Journal of Nutrition.* (2005) 93:543-547.

4. Marina, A. M., Che Man, Y. B., and Amin, I.. Virgin coconut oil: Emerging function food oil. *Trends in Food Science and Technology* 20 (2009); 481-487.

5. Remond, D., et. al. Post-prandial whole-body protein metabolism after a meat meal is influenced by chewing efficiency in the elderly subjects. *American Journal of Clinical Nutrition*, 2007; 85(5):1286-92.

6. Ceriello, A., et al. Effect of postprandial hypertriglyceridemia and hyperglycemia on circulating adhesion molecules and oxidative stress generation and the possible role of simvastatin treatment. *Diabetes* (2004); 53:701-10.

7. Nitenberg, A., et al. Postprandial endothelial dysfunction: role of glucose, lipids, and insulin. *Diabetes Metabolism* (2006); 2:2S28-33.

CHAPTER 4: MOVE TO YOUR INFLAMMATION'S CONTENT

1. L.J. Ignarro, personal communication.

2. L.J. Ignarro (ed) *Nitric Oxide Biology and Pathobiology*, San Diego, Academic Press, 2000.

3. Joseph A. Vita, Endothelial function. *Circulation*, (2011); 124:e906-912.

4. M.R. Onder and B. Barutcuoglu, *The Endothelium*, One Way Publishing, 2006.

5. Mark Houston, *Vascular Biology in Clinical Practice*, Hanley and Belfus, 2002.

6. Exposito, K., et al. Effect of weight loss and lifestyle changes on vascular inflammatory markers in obese women. *JAMA* (2003); 289:1799-1804.

7. Desouza, C.A., et al. Regular exercise prevents and restores age-related declines in endothelium-dependent vasodilatation in healthy men. *Circulation* (2000); 102:1351.

8. Wray, D.W., et al. Acute reversal of endothelial dysfunction in the elderly after antioxidant consumption. *Hypertension* (2012); 59:818-24.

CHAPTER 5: REDUCE YOUR WAIST

1. Ronti, J., et al. The endocrine function of adipose tissue: an update. *Clinical Endocrinology* (2006) 64:355-365

2. The L.E.A.N. Program, DrSearsWellnessInstitute.org

CHAPTER 6: DON'T WORRY, BE LESS INFLAMED

1. Mills, J.S. Effects of stress and uplifts on inflammation and coagulability. *Psychophysiology* (2007); 44:154-60.

2. Sapolsky, Robert M. *Why Zebras Don't Get Ulcers: An Updated Guide to Stress, Stress-Related Diseases, And Coping.* 1998, W.H. Freeman and Company.

3. Sears, William. *Prime-Time Health: A Scientifically proven Plan for Feeling Young and Living Longer.* 2010, Little, Brown and Company.

4. Selhub, Eva. M, and Logan, Alan C. *Your Brain on Nature: The Science of Nature's Influence on Your Health, Happiness, and Vitality,* 2012, Wiley.

CHAPTER 7: SELF-HELP FOR THE ABCDS: ARTHRITIS, BRONCHITIS, COLITIS, COGNITIVITIS, DERMATITIS

1. Sears, W. and Sears, M. *Prime-Time Health: a Scientifically Proven Plan for Feeling Young and Living Longer.* Little, Brown and Company, 2010.

2. Fortanasce, Vincent, David Gutkind and Robert Watkins. *End Back and Neck Pain.* Human Kinetics, 2012.

3. Fortanasce, Vincent. *The Anti-Alzheimer's Prescription.* 2008, Penguin Group (USA) Inc.

4. Perlmutter, David. *Grain Brain: The Surprising Truth about Wheat, Carbs, and Sugar – Your Brain's Silent Killers.* 2013, Little, Brown and Company.

5. Agouridis, A.P., et al. The effects of rosuvastatin alone or in combination with fenofibrate or omega-3 fatty acids, or on inflammation and oxidative stress in patients with mixed dyslipidemia. Expert Opinion in *Pharmacotherapy* 2011; 12:2605-2611.

6. Ballintyne, C.M., et al. Lipoprotein-associated phospholipase-A2, high-sensitivity C-reactive protein, and risk for incident coronary heart disease in middle-aged men and women and the

Atherosclerosis Risk in Communities (ARIC study). *Circulation* 2004; 109:837-842.

CHAPTER 8: THE INFLAMMATION SOLUTION BEGINS AT BIRTH

1. Douglas-Escobar, M. Effect of intestinal microbial ecology on the developing brain. *JAMA Pediatrics*. 2013 Apr;167(4):374-9.

2. Blaser, Martin J. *Missing Microbes*. How the overuse of antibiotics is fueling our modern Plagues, Henry Holt and Company, 2014.

3. Gregory, K., et al. Maternal breastmilk benefits establishment of preterm infant gut microbiota. Presented at Pediatric Academic Society's annual meeting, Vancouver, B.C. June 2014.

4. Sears, W., et al. *The Healthy Pregnancy Book*. Little, Brown and Company, 2013.

GRATITUDES

Thanks to those teachers who helped me grow as a doctor, author, and father. To my eight children, I give this doctorly and fatherly advice: "Surround yourselves with wise persons, and then have the wisdom and humility to listen to them." My heartfelt and healthful thanks to the following wise persons who have influenced my writings:

Dean Ornish, M.D., Founder and President of Preventive Medicine Research Institute and Clinical Professor of Medicine at the University of California, San Francisco. Reading his books, and serving with Dean on medical advisory boards, has enriched my appreciation for "doctor" first as preventer of disease, and second as prescriber of medicines.

Louis Ignarro, Ph.D., Nobel Laureate for his discovery of endothelial function. My day spent with Lou upgraded my perspective on preventive medicine when this brilliant scientist taught me the mechanism of how the body makes its own medicines.

Richard Van Praagh, M.D. Professor of Pediatrics at Harvard Medical School. Dr. Richard was my first teacher as a young intern. He instilled in me the show-me-the-science belief.

Martha Sears, R.N., M.O.M. This lovely lady in my life and mother of our eight children is my most valuable proofreader. As a tribute to our marriage, we have survived writing 42 books together. Thank you Martha!

Randy Hartnell, owner of Vital Choice Seafood Company. I respectfully call Randy "my favorite fisherman," and thank him for teaching me about the two anti-inflammatory powerhouses in wild salmon: omega-3 oils and astaxanthin.

William Harris, Ph.D. Research Professor, Sanford School of Medicine, University of South Dakota. I thank Bill for helping me understand the role of healthy and unhealthy fats in balancing, or unbalancing, inflammation.

Tracee Zeni, my reliable editorial assistant for over 23 years. Thank you, Tracee, for your diligent typing and editing of our manuscripts.

Susan Smith Jones, Ph.D., motivational speaker and author of 27 books. Thank you, Susan, for your diligent copyediting of this manuscript.

Bill Lands, Ph.D., pioneer researcher on omega balance. I thank Bill for impressing on me how omega-3/omega-6 balance affects inflammation balance.

Suzy Cohen, RPH, author of *Drug Muggers, Which Medications Are Robbing Your Body of Essential Nutrients – and Natural Ways to Restore Them*, and known as American's most trusted pharmacist. I thank you, Suzi, for impressing on me how the unhealthful side effects of anti-inflammatory drugs should motivate more people to use more skills before pills.

Gerry Cysewski, Ph.D. and Bob Capelli, two experts who taught me the inflammation balancing effects of the superfoods Hawaiian Spirulina and Astaxanthin.

Vincent Fortanasce, M.D., author of *The Anti-Alzheimer's Prescription*, Clinical Professor of Neurology at the University of Southern California, and respected godfather to two of our children. I thank Vince for helping me appreciate how inflammation is the root cause of neurodegenerative diseases.

David Katz, M.D., Founding Director of Yale University's Preventive Research Center and the Integrative Medicine Center at Griffin Hospital. I thank David for his continuing work on the NuVal® food grading system to teach consumers how proper food selection can affect inflammation.

Jeffrey Bland, Ph.D., respected as the father of functional medicine. Spending an evening at our home with Dr. Jeffrey enriched my understanding of food as medicine.

Paul Clayton, Ph.D., former Chair of the Forum on Food & Health at the Royal Society of Medicine (UK). I have the privilege of serving with Paul on a medical advisory board. I thank Paul for his insightful critique and suggestions in this book.

My wish is for you to enjoy the library of books and scientific articles written by these trusted authors.

William Sears, M.D.

INDEX